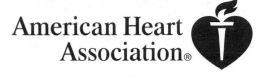

American Heart Association®

*Learn and Live*sm

Fundamentals of BLS for Healthcare Providers

Edward R. Stapleton, EMT-P, BLS Science Editor
Tom P. Aufderheide, MD, BLS Science Editor
Mary Fran Hazinski, RN, MSN, Senior ECC Science Editor
Richard O. Cummins, MD, MPH, MSc, Senior ECC Science Editor

Contributors
John M. Field, MD, ACLS Science Editor
Vinay M. Nadkarni, MD, Pediatric Science Editor
Arno Zaritsky, MD, Pediatric Science Editor
Robert A. Berg, MD
Louis Gonzales, BS, NREMT-P
Robert W. Hickey, MD
Ahamed H. Idris, MD
Graham Nichol, MD, MPH
Eric Niegelberg, NREMT-P
John Kattwinkel, MD
Richard E. Kerber, MD
Rashmi U. Kothari, MD
Peter J. Kudenchuk, MD
Susan Niermeyer, MD
Charles L. Schleien, MD
Mark E. Swanson, MD
Roger D. White, MD

International Contributors
Vic Callanan, MD
Anthony J. Handley, MD
Walter G.J. Kloeck, MD, BCh
David A. Zideman, MD

ISBN 0-87493-319-6
© 2001 American Heart Association

Contents

Preface   vii

Chapter 1
The Chain of Survival and Warning Signs of Heart Attack, Cardiac Arrest, Stroke, and Foreign-Body Airway Obstruction

Overview   1
Learning Objectives   1
Cardiovascular Disease and
   How YOU Can Help   1
AHA Adult Chain of Survival   1
   The First Link: Early Access to the
      Emergency Response System
   The Second Link: Early CPR
   The Third Link: Early Defibrillation
   The Fourth Link: Early Advanced Care
How to Recognize Life-Threatening
   Emergencies: Heart Attack,
   Cardiac Arrest, Stroke, and FBAO   4
   How to Recognize a Heart Attack
   How to Recognize Cardiac Arrest
   How to Recognize a Stroke
   How to Recognize FBAO
   Causes and Prevention of FBAO
Protecting Your Heart and Blood Vessels   10
   Major Controllable Risk Factors of
      Heart Attack and Stroke
   Are You at Risk for a Heart Attack?
Summary   13
Learning Checklist   13
Review Questions   14

Chapter 2
The ABCs of CPR: Adult CPR and Relief of FBAO

Overview   17
Learning Objectives   17
CPR: The Second Link in the
   Adult Chain of Survival   17
   The Steps of CPR
CPR Performed by 2 Rescuers   24
   Reassessment During 2-Rescuer CPR
Recovery Position   25
Face Shields, Mouth-to-Mask Devices,
   and Bag-Mask Devices   26
   Face Shields
      Using a Face Shield
   Face Masks
      Using a Face Mask
         Lateral Technique
         Cephalic Technique
   Bag-Mask Devices
      Using a Bag-Mask Device
      Cricoid Pressure (Sellick's Maneuver)
Foreign-Body Airway Obstruction   30
   First Aid for Severe or Complete FBAO
      Sequence for Relief of FBAO in the
         Responsive Victim
      Sequence for Relief of FBAO in the
         Unresponsive Victim
         Victims Who Become Unresponsive
         Victims Who Are Found Unresponsive
Keeping Your Skills Sharp: CPR Practice   33
Summary   33
Learning Checklist   33
Review Questions   34

Contents

Chapter 3
Automated External Defibrillators (AEDs)

Overview	37
Learning Objectives	37
Link Between Early Defibrillation and Survival From Cardiac Arrest	38
How AEDs Work	
How an AED Analyzes the Heart Rhythm	
Operating an AED	39
Special Conditions That Affect the Use of AEDs	
Placement of the AED	
The 4 Universal Steps of AED Operation	
Outcomes and Actions After Defibrillation	42
"Shock Indicated" Message: Recurrent VF/VT	
"No Shock Indicated"	
No Signs of Circulation	
Signs of Circulation Present	
Using AEDs in a Moving Ambulance	43
Use of an AED by 1 Rescuer	43
Integrating CPR and Use of the AED	43
When to Start CPR, When to Use the AED	
Action Sequence: The AED Protocol	
Sequence of Action for Use of an AED by 2 Rescuers	
Caring for the Victim After Successful Defibrillation	48
AED Maintenance and Troubleshooting	48
AED Treatment Algorithm	49
Summary	52
Learning Checklist	52
Review Questions	55

Chapter 4
Prevention of Injuries and Arrest in Children and Infants

Overview	57
Learning Objectives	57
AHA Chain of Survival for Infants and Children	57
Response to Cardiovascular Emergencies in Infants and Children	
Definitions of *Newly Born, Neonate, Infant, Child,* and *Adult*	
Anatomic and Physiologic Differences Affecting Cardiac Arrest and Resuscitation	
Epidemiology of Cardiopulmonary Arrest: "Phone Fast" (Infant, Child)/"Phone First" (Adult)	
BLS for Children With Special Needs	
Out-of-Hospital (EMS) Care	
Reducing the Risk of SIDS, Injury, and Arrest	61
Reducing the Risk of SIDS	
Injury: The Magnitude of the Problem	
Causes and Prevention of Common Childhood and Adolescent Injuries	
Motor Vehicle and Traffic Safety	
Passenger Injuries	
Pedestrian and Bicycle Injuries	
Submersion or Drowning	
Burns and Smoke Inhalation	
Firearm Injuries	
Poisoning	
Choking, Strangulation, and Suffocation	
Falls	
Playground Injuries	
Safety Checklist	68
Signs of Breathing Emergencies and Cardiac Arrest in Infants and Children	68
How to Recognize Breathing Emergencies	
Signs of Severe or Complete FBAO (Choking)	
Signs of Respiratory Arrest in Infants and Children	
Signs of Cardiac Arrest	
Learning Checklist	70
Review Questions	72
Safety Checklist	74

Chapter 5
The ABCs of CPR: Infant and Child CPR and Relief of Choking (FBAO)

CPR: The Second Link in the Chain of
Survival for Infants and Children   81
Learning Objectives   81
The Steps of CPR for Infants and Children   82
  1-Rescuer CPR
  2-Rescuer CPR
Recovery Position   87
Face Shields, Face Masks,
  and Bag-Mask Devices   88
  Using a Face Mask
    Lateral Technique
    Cephalic Technique
  Bag-Mask Devices
    Using a Bag-Mask Device
  Cricoid Pressure
Foreign-Body Airway Obstruction (Choking)   91
  How to Recognize Severe or Complete FBAO
    in a Responsive Infant or Child
  First Aid for Severe or Complete FBAO
    in the *Responsive* Infant or Child
    Relief of Complete FBAO in a Responsive Infant
    Relief of Complete FBAO in a Responsive Child
  Sequence for Relief of FBAO in an
    Unresponsive Infant or Child
    Victims Who Become Unresponsive
    Victims Who Are Found Unresponsive
Presence of Victim's Family Members
  During Resuscitation   95
Stopping Resuscitative Efforts   95
Summary   96
Learning Checklist   96
Review Questions   98

Chapter 6
Special Resuscitation Situations

Overview   101
Learning Objectives   101
Hypothermia   101
  Basic Life Support
Submersion/Near-Drowning   103
  Rescue From the Water
  Rescue Breathing
  Chest Compressions and Defibrillation
Cardiac Arrest Associated With Trauma   104
  Extrication and Initial Evaluation
  Establish Unresponsiveness
  Airway
  Breathing/Ventilation
  Circulation
  Disability
  Exposure
Electric Shock and Lightning Strike   105
  Electric Shock
  Lightning Strike
  Modifications of BLS for Arrest Caused by
    Electric Shock or Lightning Strike
Pregnancy   106
Allergies   106
Asphyxia   106
Exceptions to "Phone First" for
  Unresponsive Adults   107
Summary   107
Learning Checklist   107
Review Questions   108

Chapter 7
Safety During CPR Training and Actual Rescue

Overview	111
Learning Objectives	111
Disease Transmission During CPR Training	111
Disease Transmission During Actual Performance of CPR	112
Barrier Devices: Face Masks and Face Shields	113
Summary	113
Learning Checklist	113
Review Questions	114

Chapter 8
The Human Dimension of CPR: Psychosocial and Legal Issues

Outcomes of Resuscitation Attempts: Definitions of "Success"	117
Learning Objectives	117
Stress Reactions	117
Techniques to Prevent and Reduce Stress in Rescuers, Families, and Witnesses	
Critical Incident Stress Debriefings	
Psychological Barriers to Action	118
Legal Aspects of CPR	119
"Good Samaritan" Immunity for CPR Performed in the Community	
Decisions About Resuscitation	
Determination of Death Outside the Hospital	
Discontinuation of Resuscitation in Hospitals	
CPR in Nursing Homes	
Community Systems for Communicating No-CPR Orders	
Summary	120
Learning Checklist	121
Review Questions	121

Appendix A
Comparison Across Age Groups of Resuscitation Interventions

	123

Appendix B
Skills Performance Sheets

	125
Adult 1-Rescuer CPR	127
Adult Bag-Mask Ventilation	128
Adult 2-Rescuer CPR	129
Adult FBAO in Responsive Victim	130
Adult FBAO in Unresponsive Victim	131
Infant 1-Rescuer CPR	132
Infant Bag-Mask Ventilation	133
Infant FBAO in Responsive Victim	134
Infant FBAO in Unresponsive Victim	135
Infant and Child 2-Rescuer CPR	136
Child 1-Rescuer CPR	137
Child Bag-Mask Ventilation	138
Child FBAO in Responsive Victim	139
Child FBAO in Unresponsive Victim	140
CPR and AED Performance Criteria for Victims 1 to 8 Years of Age	141
Integrated Adult FBAO and Rescue Breathing — Performance Evaluation	143
Integrated Infant FBAO, CPR, and Rescue Breathing — Performance Evaluation	144
Integrated Child FBAO, CPR, and Rescue Breathing — Performance Evaluation	146
Adult 1- and 2-Rescuer CPR With AED — Performance Evaluation	148

Glossary

	149

Preface

The AHA offers a variety of courses on basic life support (BLS) and cardiopulmonary resuscitation (CPR) for healthcare providers. With the knowledge and skills you learn in these courses, you can save the life of a family member, a friend, a coworker, a citizen in your community, or a patient in the hospital or clinic where you work.

The BLS for Healthcare Providers Course is intended for participants who must have a credential (a card) documenting successful completion of a course in CPR and BLS for healthcare professionals. Such credentials are typically required for people who provide healthcare to patients in a wide variety of settings, both in-hospital and outside the hospital.

This course will teach you how to recognize and respond to life-threatening emergencies such as cardiac arrest, respiratory arrest, and foreign-body airway obstruction (choking). You will learn to recognize heart attack and stroke in adults and breathing difficulty in children. This course teaches the skills needed to respond to the emergencies you identify. You will learn the skills of CPR for victims of all ages (including ventilation with barrier devices and bag-mask devices), use of an automated external defibrillator (AED), and relief of foreign body airway obstruction. These skills will enable you to recognize emergencies and provide the first three links in either the AHA adult Chain of Survival or the pediatric Chain of Survival. With these skills you may save the life of a patient, a member of your community, or a loved one.

Participants in this course will use one of two manuals, *BLS for Healthcare Providers* or this manual, *Fundamentals of BLS for Healthcare Providers.*

BLS for Healthcare Providers is intended for use by licensed and certified healthcare professionals. It assumes that the reader has a healthcare education, and it contains a stronger emphasis on anatomy and physiology and on scientific rationale for actions and recommendations than is included in *Fundamentals of BLS*. You will also find information about reducing risk of heart disease and injury prevention that you may wish to use for patient education.

This manual is designed to provide information that will be useful to you before, during and after the BLS for Healthcare Providers Course. It contains several features designed to help you learn CPR, ventilation with a barrier device and a bag-mask device, and use of an AED. Each chapter includes *learning objectives,* a *learning checklist,* and *review questions.* These features will make learning easier. At the start of each chapter, carefully read the learning objectives. Reading them carefully will help you focus on the essential information. When you finish reading the chapter, review the learning checklist. Then answer the review questions. If you cannot answer a question or if you choose the wrong answer, review the parts of the chapter related to that question.

Throughout the manual you will see colored boxes. These boxes highlight important and useful information. **Critical Concepts** presents essential information for mastering the knowledge and skills taught in this course. Critical signs and symptoms included in these boxes and in the text are called **red flags.** A **red flag** says "Warning! This is vital information about critical signs and symptoms."

Foundation Facts further explains the recommended actions and provide important supportive information.

FYI boxes present background material for your information only. These boxes contain information about various topics, such as different types of 911 systems, that may be useful or interesting to some participants. You are *not required* to know the information presented in FYI boxes to fulfill the core learning objectives.

The skills performance sheets ("Performance Criteria") in the appendix of this manual list the skills you will practice in class. To obtain a course completion card, you must satisfactorily demonstrate the skills listed on each sheet to your instructor, and you must score at least 84% on a written examination. Review each skill, read each chapter in this manual, pay attention to the details, and practice carefully. It is easy to forget some CPR skills, so practice the skills and reread this manual after you complete the course.

The appendix also contains case scenarios. These scenarios will help you learn to apply your knowledge of CPR to realistic situations. Take advantage of this learning opportunity. It will do more than prepare you for the course. It will prepare you to save a life.

To obtain more information about ways to reduce the risk of heart disease, stroke, and injury and updated information on CPR, visit the AHA website at www.americanheart.org/cpr. This site also contains links to other sites with useful information.

This printing of the text includes new recommendations regarding use of AEDs in children published by the AHA in association with the International Liaison Committee on Resuscitation (ILCOR) in July, 2003. For more information you can find the full text of the recommendation and other information related to CPR and ECC at www.americanheart.org/cpr.

We wish you success as you learn CPR. When you complete the course, you will be prepared to recognize emergencies in adults, to prevent many causes of cardiac arrest in infants and children, and to respond to emergencies using the skills of CPR.

Edward R. Stapleton, EMT-P

Tom P. Aufderheide, MD

Mary Fran Hazinski, RN, MSN

You work in a long-term care facility, where you help care for a 65-year-old man. You go into his room to pick up his dinner tray and find him clutching his chest. He is pale and sweaty. He says he has had discomfort in his chest for 30 minutes and that the pain has traveled to his jaw and down his left arm. He has no history of heart disease. You phone the emergency response number at the facility and, according to protocol, administer oxygen at a rate of 4 L/min.

The medical director arrives and examines the patient, and she agrees that the patient may be having a heart attack (myocardial infarction). You help transport the patient to a local hospital capable of providing care for patients with acute coronary syndromes. Before leaving for the hospital, you notify the hospital Emergency Department (ED) that you will be arriving by ambulance with a victim of potential myocardial infarction. You obtain a 12-lead electrocardiogram and transmit the results to the hospital.

The ED triage nurse greets you and your patient when you arrive, and your patient is immediately evaluated. The patient receives fibrinolytic therapy and is discharged back to the healthcare facility 5 days later with a favorable prognosis. When you next care for him, he thanks you for your persistent and thoughtful care.

The Chain of Survival and Warning Signs of Heart Attack, Cardiac Arrest, Stroke, and Foreign-Body Airway Obstruction

Overview

What are the signs of heart attack, stroke, cardiac arrest, and foreign-body airway obstruction (FBAO) (that is, choking) in adults? Why is early recognition so critical to these patients? Why is it important to phone the emergency response number as soon as you detect signs of heart attack or stroke? After reading this chapter, you will be able to answer these questions and more.

Cardiovascular Disease and How YOU Can Help

Cardiovascular disease is the leading cause of death in the United States. Every year more than 529,000 adult Americans die of a heart attack or related complications. About half of these deaths (250,000) result from sudden cardiac arrest. Sudden cardiac arrest occurs when the heart suddenly stops beating. Most often it is caused by an arrhythmia (an abnormal heart rhythm) called *ventricular fibrillation* (VF) that prevents the heart from pumping blood.

Sudden cardiac arrest can complicate a heart attack. Sudden cardiac arrest is most likely to occur during the *first hour* after the onset of symptoms of a heart attack, typically before the victim arrives at the hospital. Sudden cardiac arrest will result in death unless emergency treatments, including cardiopulmonary resuscitation (CPR) and defibrillation, are provided immediately. Although CPR doubles the victim's chance of survival, the definitive treatment for VF is *defibrillation* with a medical device called a *defibrillator*. Some computerized defibrillators, called automated external defibrillators (AEDs), can be used by healthcare providers and lay rescuers alike.

The victim of an emergency such as a heart attack, cardiac arrest, stroke, or FBAO (choking) can be saved if people at the scene begin the Chain of Survival. In this chapter you will learn the critical actions that comprise

<table>
<tr><td>

Learning Objectives

After reading this chapter you will be able to

1. Name the links in the AHA adult Chain of Survival and discuss the role you play in the Chain of Survival

2. List the warning signs of 4 major emergencies in adults:

   ■ Heart attack

   ■ Cardiac arrest

   ■ Stroke

   ■ Foreign-body airway obstruction (choking)

</td></tr>
</table>

the 4 links in the American Heart Association (AHA) adult Chain of Survival. You will learn how to recognize the symptoms of a heart attack, cardiac arrest, stroke, and FBAO (choking). You will learn when to phone the emergency response number at your workplace (or 911), when and how to perform CPR and defibrillation, and when and how to relieve FBAO in adults.

AHA Adult Chain of Survival

The AHA adult Chain of Survival symbol (Figure 1) depicts the critical actions required to treat life-threatening emergencies, including heart attack, cardiac arrest, stroke, and FBAO (choking).

Once you recognize an emergency, *immediately* provide

■ **Early access to the emergency response system** in your healthcare facility or community to ensure that additional rescuers and those capable of providing advanced life support arrive as quickly as possible.

- **Early CPR** to support circulation to the heart and brain until normal heart activity is restored.

- **Early defibrillation** to treat cardiac arrest caused by VF.

Early advanced care will be provided by EMS and hospital personnel with additional training and expertise.

You must know when to activate the Chain of Survival. You must recognize when an emergency exists. At the end of this course you will have the knowledge and skills needed to complete 3 of the 4 links in the Chain of Survival. When you recognize an emergency and phone the emergency response number, begin CPR, and use an AED, *you* are performing the actions that increase a victim's chance of survival. Skilled rescuers and healthcare professionals will respond to the emergency call. They will be trained and equipped to provide defibrillation (if it was unavailable to you) and advanced care to further increase the victim's chance of survival.

To save people with heart attack, cardiac arrest, or stroke, *each set of actions or link in the Chain of Survival must be performed as soon as possible.* If any link in the chain is weak, delayed, or missing, the victim's chance of survival decreases. The following sections describe each link in the Chain of Survival

The First Link: Early Access to the Emergency Response System

The first step in the treatment of any emergency is recognizing that an emergency exists and phoning the appropriate emergency response number. A healthcare facility may have an internal number (hospital extension) that activates the emergency response team. In the community 911 is the most common emergency response number.

You must recognize the warning signs of a heart attack, cardiac arrest, stroke, or FBAO (choking). *Anyone who is unresponsive* should receive emergency care. Heart attack, cardiac arrest, stroke, and FBAO can cause unresponsiveness. Although many other conditions can cause unresponsiveness, *all* victims who suddenly become unresponsive will benefit from activation of the Chain of Survival.

In most healthcare settings an emergency response team is available on-site to respond quickly to emergencies. If such a response team is on-site, healthcare providers should contact that system instead of the EMS system (911). The operator who answers your call will determine your location and the nature of the emergency, notify the emergency response team, and send other trained rescuers to help you. If you work in a facility with an internal emergency response team, whenever this manual states "phone 911," you should phone the emergency response number at your workplace.

Your workplace may have AEDs available for use by you and other healthcare providers. If AEDs are available, the rescuer who phones the emergency response number should get the AED (usually located near the phone).

AEDs are also becoming more commonplace in public settings such as malls, airports, and casinos. As a healthcare provider trained in CPR and the use of AEDs, you may have the opportunity to save someone in your community. In most states healthcare providers and lay rescuers who function as "Good Samaritans" are provided limited immunity (legal protection) when they use an AED to help a victim of cardiac arrest outside a healthcare facility.

Often in an emergency you are not alone with the victim. Other rescuers or bystanders are nearby. If you find a person who is unresponsive, shout for help to bring other rescuers to help you. Then send another rescuer to phone the emergency response number while you begin CPR.

When you phone the emergency response number, the operator or dispatcher will ask questions and relay the

FIGURE 1. The AHA adult Chain of Survival. The 4 links or sets of actions in the chain are **(1)** early access to the emergency response system, **(2)** early CPR, **(3)** early defibrillation, and **(4)** early advanced care.

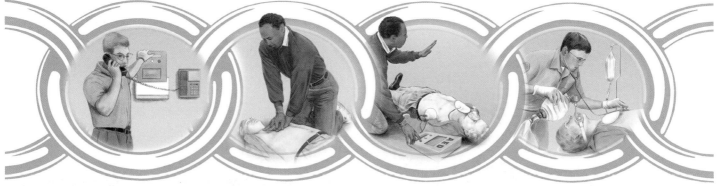

information you provide to the emergency response team. Give short, specific answers. Give only the requested information. The dispatcher will probably ask the following questions:

- **"What is your emergency?"** You might answer: *"The patient in the CT scanner complained of chest pain and became unresponsive."*

- **"What's happening now?"** *"The lab tech is beginning CPR, and I'm getting the AED."*

- **"Where is the victim located?"** *"We're in CT scanner room B on the first floor in Diagnostic Radiology."*

- **"What number are you calling from?"** *"Extension 2-1313."*

At this point the operator will give you directions or ask more questions.

The Second Link: Early CPR

CPR is a set of actions that the rescuer performs in sequence to *assess and support* airway, breathing, and circulation as needed. CPR is performed in steps (Figure 2) so that the rescuer provides only the support the victim needs.

CPR is the critical link that buys time between the first link (early access to the emergency response system) and the third link (early defibrillation). CPR supports delivery of oxygen to the brain and heart until defibrillation or other advanced care can restore normal heart action. *Victims of out-of-hospital cardiac arrest who receive CPR from bystanders are more than twice as likely to survive as victims who do not receive CPR.* The earlier you give CPR to a person in cardiac or respiratory arrest, the greater the victim's chance of survival.

The Third Link: Early Defibrillation

Most adult victims of witnessed sudden cardiac arrest are in VF. VF is an abnormal, chaotic heart rhythm that prevents the heart from pumping blood.

The treatment for VF is *defibrillation*. Defibrillation is the delivery of a shock to the heart that stops VF and allows a normal heart rhythm to resume. When VF occurs, prompt defibrillation will increase the victim's chance of survival. With each minute that defibrillation is delayed, the victim's chance of survival falls by 7% to 10%. If defibrillation is performed within the first 5 minutes of cardiac arrest caused by VF, the victim's chance of survival is about 50%. After 10 to 12 minutes of cardiac arrest, there is little chance of survival *unless CPR has been provided.* CPR prolongs the time that defibrillation can be effective. To increase the victim's chance of survival, you must provide CPR until defibrillation is performed.

Medical care facilities may have manual defibrillators, AEDs, or both. AEDs can be used to deliver a shock to the victim in cardiac arrest before the arrival of rescuers who can provide advanced care. If an AED is available, get the AED when you phone 911 (or other emergency response number). Then you or others trained in the use of AEDs will be able to provide early defibrillation if needed. Every medical professional must know how to operate an AED.

An AED is attached to the victim with 2 adhesive electrode pads. The AED analyzes the rhythm of the victim's heart, determines if a shock is needed, and charges to the appropriate dose of energy. The rescuer presses a SHOCK button to deliver the shock when prompted by the AED.

FIGURE 2. The steps of CPR. CPR includes both assessment and support steps, performed in sequence. The rescuer provides only the support the victim needs.

Reassess

Continue "pump and blow" for 1 minute

If no signs of circulation: begin chest compressions

Assess for signs of circulation

If no breathing: give 2 rescue breaths

Open the airway: look, listen, and feel for breathing

If no response: phone 911

Assess responsiveness

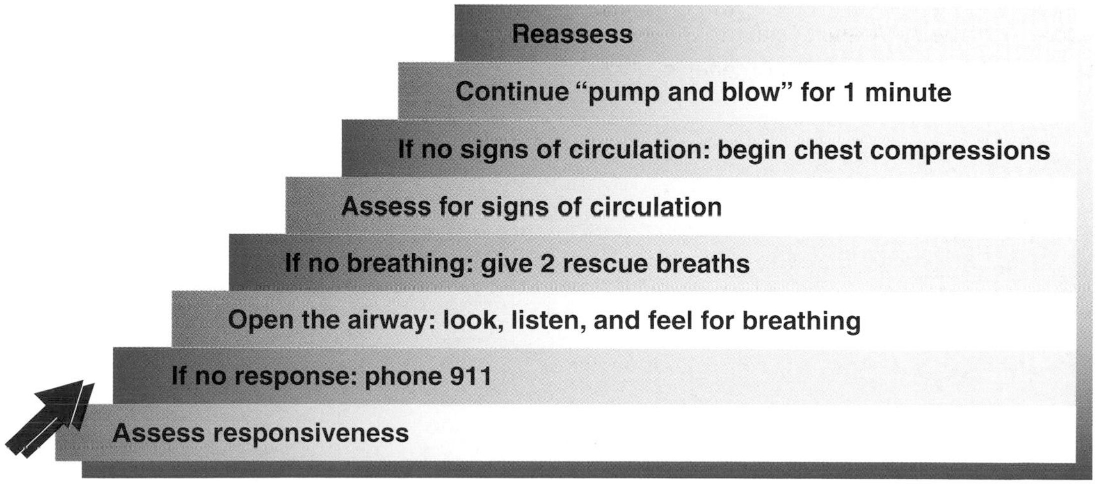

This course will provide you with the knowledge and skills needed to use an AED. Chapter 3 of this manual describes use of an AED in more detail. Remember to ask your employer if an AED is available for your use and if a protocol exists for its use. Also check your state's laws on use of AEDs in public access defibrillation (PAD programs).

The Fourth Link: Early Advanced Care

The fourth link in the AHA adult Chain of Survival is early advanced care. Highly trained EMS personnel called *paramedics* provide advanced care outside the hospital. Inside the hospital teams of highly skilled providers of advanced cardiovascular life support (ACLS) give advanced care to victims of cardiac arrest.

Advanced care includes the administration of drugs and insertion of breathing (tracheal) tubes to (1) help the heart in VF respond to defibrillation, (2) maintain a normal rhythm after successful defibrillation, and (3) support oxygenation and ventilation. ACLS also includes use of numerous assessments and interventions to treat noncardiac causes of respiratory and cardiac arrest. You can learn ACLS skills in the AHA Advanced Cardiovascular Life Support Course.

FYI: AEDs and PAD Programs

Automated external defibrillators (AEDs) are computerized defibrillators that may be safely operated by healthcare providers and lay rescuers who have only a few hours of training. AEDs are extremely accurate and relatively inexpensive. They can reduce the time to defibrillation if they are available to trained rescuers who use them before EMS or advanced healthcare personnel arrive.

Lay rescuer AED programs are a public health initiative developed by the AHA. Lay rescuer AED programs are designed to increase the number of AEDs available in a community and to increase the number of rescuers trained to provide CPR and use an AED.

AEDs can be used in the community by "Good Samaritan" healthcare providers, firefighters, police officers, airline personnel, and trained lay rescuers before EMS personnel arrive. AEDs will reduce the time to defibrillation if they are used before EMS personnel arrive. Prompt defibrillation increases the victim's chance of survival from cardiac arrest.

In this course you will be trained to provide CPR and operate an AED.

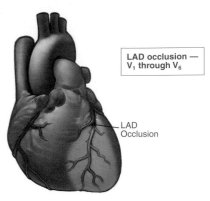

FIGURE 3. Blocked coronary artery. LAD indicates left anterior descending artery.

LAD occlusion — V_1 through V_6

LAD Occlusion

How to Recognize Life-Threatening Emergencies: Heart Attack, Cardiac Arrest, Stroke, and FBAO

How to Recognize a Heart Attack

A heart attack occurs when the heart muscle does not receive enough oxygen and heart muscle starts to die. A heart attack is caused by blockage in a coronary artery, one of the major blood vessels that supplies blood and oxygen to the heart muscle (Figure 3). *Acute myocardial infarction* is the medical term for heart attack. New drugs called clotbusters can unblock the coronary arteries of some patients if they are given within a few hours of the onset of signs of a heart attack.

The most important and most common symptom of a heart attack is chest discomfort, pressure, or pain. The pain develops in the center of the chest, behind the breastbone (sternum). The pain may travel to the neck, jaw, or down the arm (usually the left arm). It usually lasts more than 3 to 5 minutes. **Chest pain** is a *red flag*. The flag says *Warning! Think heart attack.*

A person having a heart attack is usually awake and can talk but feels uncomfortable or is in pain. Time is critical. Clotbusters are most effective when given within 90 minutes after symptoms of a heart attack begin. If you think someone is having a heart attack, immediately activate the emergency response system (phone 911 or other emergency response number). Minutes count! Know the symptoms!

If you see someone with chest discomfort and you think the person is having a heart attack, ask these questions:

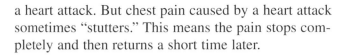

■ **"What is the pain like?"** People describe the discomfort caused by a heart attack in many ways: as a pressure, fullness, squeezing, pain, or heaviness. The person may not feel pain but may say he or she feels pressure or *discomfort* in the chest. The discomfort may or may not be severe.

■ **"Where is the pain located?"** People usually feel the discomfort right behind the breastbone, deep in the center of the chest (Figure 4). After a few moments the pain may spread to the shoulder, neck, lower jaw, or arm. The pain may be on the left side, right side, or both sides, but often it is located on the left side. Sometimes the pain or discomfort may be felt even in the back, between the shoulder blades.

■ **"How long have you had the pain?"** The discomfort of a heart attack usually lasts more than a few minutes. Sharp, stabbing, knifelike pain that lasts only a second and then disappears is usually not the pain of

FIGURE 4. Typical locations of chest pain caused by a heart attack.

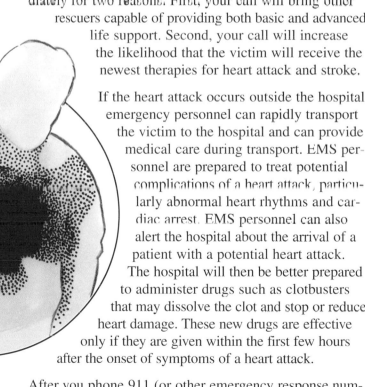

a heart attack. But chest pain caused by a heart attack sometimes "stutters." This means the pain stops completely and then returns a short time later.

Not all warning signs occur in every heart attack. People who are having a heart attack may have vague signs. They may say they feel lightheaded, faint, short of breath, or nauseous. They may describe their chest discomfort as an ache, heartburn, or indigestion. Other signs include sweating, nausea, vomiting, or shortness of breath. These vague signs of a heart attack are more common in women, people with diabetes, and the elderly.

Many people will not admit that they may be having a heart attack. People react with a variety of statements or excuses. They may say "I'm too healthy," "I don't want to bother the doctor," "I don't want to frighten my wife," "I'll feel ridiculous if it isn't a heart attack," or "I hate red lights and sirens."

When a person with symptoms of a heart attack tries to downplay what he or she is feeling, *you* must take responsibility and act at once. Tell the victim to sit quietly. Phone the emergency response number (or 911) and get the AED. Be prepared to perform CPR.

You must phone the emergency response number immediately for two reasons. First, your call will bring other rescuers capable of providing both basic and advanced life support. Second, your call will increase the likelihood that the victim will receive the newest therapies for heart attack and stroke.

If the heart attack occurs outside the hospital, emergency personnel can rapidly transport the victim to the hospital and can provide medical care during transport. EMS personnel are prepared to treat potential complications of a heart attack, particularly abnormal heart rhythms and cardiac arrest. EMS personnel can also alert the hospital about the arrival of a patient with a potential heart attack. The hospital will then be better prepared to administer drugs such as clotbusters that may dissolve the clot and stop or reduce heart damage. These new drugs are effective only if they are given within the first few hours after the onset of symptoms of a heart attack.

After you phone 911 (or other emergency response number), have the person rest quietly and calmly. Help the person into a position that is comfortable and that allows the easiest breathing.

FYI: Emergency Medical Dispatch Assistance and Enhanced 911

In many areas of the United States emergency medical dispatchers (EMDs) are taught how to help callers give emergency care. The instructions are simple, and they will help you help the victim until EMS personnel arrive. Remember, early access to the emergency response system (phoning 911 or other emergency response number), early CPR, and early defibrillation with an AED are 3 critical links in the Chain of Survival that you *must perform immediately* to increase the victim's chances of survival.

Using a prepared list of instructions, the EMD will coach you through the basic steps of CPR and operation of an AED. If you can bring the phone to the victim's side, follow the dispatcher's instructions. If other rescuers are at the scene and the EMD provides instructions, remain on the telephone and do the following:

■ Repeat the dispatcher's instructions loudly to the other rescuers and confirm that the rescuers are following each step.

■ Tell the dispatcher if the victim vomits or other complications occur. Rescuers are not expected to perform perfectly in such a crisis.

■ Ensure that rescuers follow each instruction, even if it takes extra seconds.

■ Ensure the safety of the rescuers at all times.

■ When EMS personnel arrive at the victim's side, the dispatcher will hang up after confirming their arrival.

■ You hang up last. Stay on the line until the dispatcher hangs up or instructs you to do so. The dispatcher will hang up after confirming arrival of EMS personnel at the victim's side.

■ Find out if your community has **enhanced 911.** Enhanced 911 operates in a manner similar to "caller ID." With enhanced 911 systems a computer automatically confirms the caller's *address* and phone number. This allows the dispatcher to locate the caller even if the caller is unable to speak or the connection is broken. If your community does not have enhanced 911, become a vocal advocate for such services in your community. Enhanced 911 can save precious seconds, minutes, and lives.

Critical Concepts: Red Flags of a Heart Attack

People who are having a heart attack may have several or few warning signs, or they may have only vague signs. If *any* signs occur, don't wait. Get help immediately. Phone 911 or the emergency response number. Delay can be deadly.

Red flags of a heart attack include

■ Chest *discomfort, pressure, or pain*

■ *Lightheadedness* or "feeling dizzy" during the pain.

■ *Fainting* or loss of responsiveness

■ *Sweating* or "breaking out in a cold sweat all over" but without fever

■ *Nausea*, usually without vomiting

■ *Shortness of breath,* especially worrisome if the victim is short of breath during the pain, while lying still or resting, or when moving only a little

How to Recognize Cardiac Arrest

In cardiac arrest blood flow stops and the brain, heart, and other organs are deprived of oxygen. The victim will be unresponsive and will have no adequate breathing, no signs of circulation, and no pulse. The victim will have no signs of circulation (no adequate breathing, coughing, or movement) in response to rescue breaths.

Victims in cardiac arrest often gasp for breath. These gasps are called agonal respirations. They may occur early in cardiac arrest, and they are *not* effective breaths. Agonal respirations will not maintain oxygenation or ventilation, so a victim who is gasping is *not* breathing adequately.

Both healthcare providers and lay rescuers assess for breathing as a sign of circulation. Lay rescuers are generally taught to look for "normal" breathing. Healthcare providers should be able to distinguish between adequate and inadequate breathing, and they should provide rescue breathing if the victim's breathing is inadequate. Healthcare providers should also recognize agonal respirations.

Sudden unresponsiveness is a red flag of cardiac arrest. Act immediately! The victim of cardiac arrest will have **3 red flags:**

1. **No response:** Victims of cardiac arrest do not respond when you speak to or touch them. If you are alone

Critical Concepts:
Red Flags of Cardiac Arrest

The victim in cardiac arrest has the following red flags:

- No response
- No adequate breathing
- No signs of circulation (no breathing, coughing, or movement)

with someone who suddenly becomes unresponsive, immediately phone 911 or other emergency response number. If a second rescuer is present, send that rescuer to phone 911 and get the AED while you begin CPR.

2. **No adequate breathing:** Once you discover that the victim is unresponsive and the emergency response number has been called, begin CPR. Open the airway and look, listen, and feel for breathing. Victims of cardiac arrest do not breathe adequately. Give the victim 2 rescue breaths.

3. **No signs of circulation:** After you give 2 breaths to the victim, check for signs of circulation. Look for a response to the 2 breaths. If the heart is beating and delivering oxygen to the brain and body, the victim will respond to the 2 breaths. The response will be adequate breathing, coughing, or movement. Check for signs of circulation for no more than 10 seconds.

   - Put your head near the victim's nose and mouth, open the airway, and look, listen, and feel for breathing. Take about 5 seconds.
   - Look at the victim's body for coughing or movement.
   - If you do not see signs of circulation, begin chest compressions.

The steps of CPR are summarized in Chapter 2.

Critical Concepts:
Critical Actions to Take if You Are Alone

If you are alone and find someone who is unresponsive:

- Phone 911 (or other emergency response number) and get the AED
- Begin CPR if needed

FYI: Heart Rhythms That Cause Cardiac Arrest

Cardiac arrest can be caused by the following heart rhythms:

- Ventricular fibrillation (VF)
- Ventricular tachycardia (VT)
- Pulseless electrical activity
- Asystole

VF is an abnormal rhythm that causes the heart muscle to quiver. This quivering prevents the heart from pumping blood. VT is a very rapid rhythm. The rhythm can be so rapid that the heart does not pump enough blood to create a pulse. VF and "pulseless" VT can develop as complications of a heart attack, even in men or women who have no chest pain. VF and sudden cardiac arrest may be the first and *only* signs of a heart attack in some victims. VT and pulseless VT are treated with defibrillation. Asystole and pulseless electrical activity are treated with CPR and advanced life support.

FYI: Respiratory Arrest

Respiratory arrest is present when the victim is not breathing at all or is breathing so slowly, shallowly, or irregularly that oxygenation of the blood cannot occur. The term *respiratory arrest* is used for victims who are not breathing adequately but who *still have signs of circulation.*

You will identify respiratory arrest as you perform the steps of CPR. A victim of respiratory arrest will be unresponsive. Open the airway and look, listen, and feel for breathing. You will observe no breathing or only occasional or very shallow breaths. Such breathing will not deliver oxygen to the brain and other organs. Give 2 breaths, watching the chest to see if it rises with each breath.

The victim in respiratory arrest will have signs of circulation (breathing, coughing, or movement) in response to the rescue breaths. These signs confirm that the victim has spontaneous blood flow (circulation) and that cardiac arrest is *not* present. If the victim does not have normal, adequate breathing, *respiratory arrest* is present. These victims require rescue breathing (give 1 breath every 5 seconds).

Case Scenario

You are performing a home health visit for an elderly woman with hypertension and diabetes. When you arrive her husband tells you that 20 minutes ago his wife began slurring her words. Since then she has been unable to get up from her chair because of weakness in her left leg. You observe no problems with airway, breathing, or circulation, so you quickly assess the woman using the Cincinnati Stroke Scale.

You identify a droop on the right side of her face, weakness in the left arm, and slurring of speech. You strongly suspect a stroke. According to what the husband has told you, the symptoms began at 2:50 pm (27 minutes ago). Both the wife and husband ask you to drive them to the community hospital close to their home. You quickly explain the importance of early activation of the EMS system and then phone 911.

You tell the dispatcher you suspect that your patient has had a stroke. An EMS team arrives within a few minutes. They perform a stroke assessment, and they agree that your patient has probably had a stroke. The EMS team notifies the nearest hospital capable of providing acute stroke care that they are transporting the patient to that hospital. A stroke team is waiting for the patient when she arrives at the hospital at 3:30 pm (40 minutes after the onset of stroke symptoms).

The husband calls you 2 days later to thank you. He says his wife received fibrinolytic therapy shortly after she arrived at the hospital and that all her symptoms have resolved.

FIGURE 5. Facial droop in a victim of stroke. **A,** Normal. **B,** Facial droop.

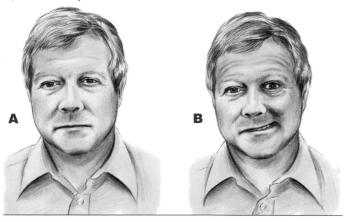

How to Recognize a Stroke

A stroke is the rapid onset of neurologic problems. A stroke can develop when a blood vessel in the brain becomes blocked so that an area of the brain receives no blood and no oxygen, or it can develop when a blood vessel in the brain ruptures and bleeds into the brain. Stroke is a leading cause of death and serious disability among Americans. Although most strokes occur in older people, *strokes can occur in people of all ages.*

Signs of stroke include (1) sudden numbness or weakness of face, arm, or leg, especially on one side of the body, (2) sudden confusion, trouble speaking or understanding, (3) sudden trouble seeing in one or both eyes, (4) sudden trouble walking, dizziness, loss of balance or coordination, or (5) sudden severe headache with no known cause.

Strokes sometimes damage areas of the brain that control breathing, and they may cause the victim to become unresponsive. If this occurs the victim may stop breathing or may develop airway obstruction. If these complications develop, you will need to perform some or all of the steps of CPR, particularly rescue breathing. Although breathing difficulty or respiratory arrest may develop as a complication of stroke, cardiac arrest does not often occur with a stroke in the out-of-hospital setting.

You must know the **signs of stroke** so that you can phone the emergency response number (or 911). Many signs of stroke are vague or ignored by the victim. If you think someone has had a stroke, look closely for the sudden onset of one of these *red flags:*

1. **Facial droop:** This sign is most obvious if the victim smiles or grimaces. If one side of the face droops or the face does not move (Figure 5), a stroke may have occurred.

2. **Arm weakness:** This sign is most obvious if the victim extends his arms with the eyes closed (Figure 6). If one arm drifts downward or the victim cannot move his arms, a stroke may have occurred.

3. **Speech difficulties:** The victim is unable to talk or will slur words. Ask the victim to repeat a sentence such as "You can't teach an old dog new tricks." If the victim cannot repeat the sentence accurately and clearly, a stroke may have occurred.

Whenever you think someone is having a stroke, phone the emergency response number (or 911) immediately! If you are in a medical facility, shout for help immediately (other rescuers are likely to be nearby). The victim of stroke requires immediate medical evaluation and may be eligible for new therapies to reduce injury to the brain. If the victim is outside a medical facility, EMS personnel will examine and quickly transport the victim to a hospital for evaluation and treatment.

New and effective treatments for stroke are now available, but they must be given *within the first 3 hours* after the onset of signs of a stroke. These drugs include clot-busters (fibrinolytic agents) that may reduce the disability caused by a stroke. Because the time for administration of these new stroke treatments is limited, the victim must be *immediately* evaluated in a hospital capable of providing acute stroke care.

If you think someone is having a stroke, don't wait. Phone 911 immediately. EMS personnel can evaluate the victim, transport the victim to the hospital, support the victim during transport, and notify the hospital of the victim's condition before arrival. This will ensure that the victim receives rapid evaluation and therapy.

To help treat a victim of stroke, you must

- Recognize the signs of stroke

- Access the emergency response system (call 911 or other emergency response number)

- Perform CPR if needed (opening the airway may be all that is needed in the unresponsive victim)

Family members and bystanders often fail to phone 911 when a stroke occurs. Do not assume that the stroke victim's symptoms are caused by alcohol or drug intoxication or medical conditions such as low blood sugar. *If you think a person is having a stroke, do not delay: Phone 911 or other emergency response number immediately.*

FIGURE 6. Arm weakness in a victim of stroke. **A,** Normal. **B,** Arm weakness.

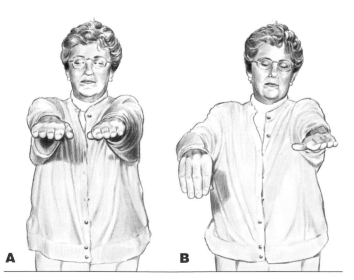

A   **B**

Critical Concepts: Red Flags of Stroke

Cincinnati Stroke Scale

The *sudden* onset of

1. Facial droop
2. Arm weakness
3. Speech difficulties

How to Recognize FBAO

Every year FBAO (choking) causes about 3000 deaths in the United States. FBAO in adults usually occurs during eating. Poorly chewed meat is the most frequent cause of choking in adults, but a variety of foods and foreign bodies can obstruct the airway.

Foreign bodies may *partially* block the airway but still allow adequate air movement. Choking victims with only *partial obstruction* of the airway will be responsive and will cough forcefully. Usually they can speak. Their breath sounds may be noisy. These victims require no immediate action from you, but be prepared to act if the obstruction becomes severe or complete.

You do *not* need to act if the choking victim can cough forcefully and speak. A victim who can cough and speak has only *partial* obstruction of the airway and is able to move air. **Do not interfere** at this point because a strong cough is the most effective way to remove a foreign body. Stay with the victim and monitor his or her condition. If the partial obstruction persists, phone 911 or other emergency response number.

Victims with *severe or complete* FBAO will initially be responsive but will not be able to move enough air to cough forcefully or speak. They may make high-pitched noises when they try to inhale. If severe or complete FBAO is present, give abdominal thrusts (the Heimlich maneuver) to relieve the obstruction.

To treat airway obstruction successfully, *you must first recognize it.* If a foreign body is completely obstructing the airway, remove it. Review the Critical Concepts box to remember the *red flags* of severe FBAO.

Causes and Prevention of FBAO

The best way to treat FBAO (choking) is to prevent it. Factors that contribute to choking in adults include

- Swallowing large, poorly chewed pieces of food

- Eating after drinking alcoholic beverages (eating while under the influence of alcohol can lead to swallowing large pieces of food)

Critical Concepts: Red Flags of Severe FBAO

- Universal sign of choking (hands clutching the throat) (Figure 7)

- Ask "Are you choking?" If the victim nods, ask "Can you speak?" If the victim cannot speak, the airway obstruction is severe or complete.

- Weak, ineffective, or silent coughs

- High-pitched sounds or no sounds while inhaling

- Increased difficulty breathing

- Blue lips or skin (cyanosis)

- Wearing dentures

- Playing, crying, laughing, or talking while food or foreign bodies are in the mouth

To prevent choking:

- Cut food into small pieces and chew them slowly and thoroughly, especially if you wear dentures

- Avoid excessive intake of alcohol, particularly while eating

- Avoid laughing and talking while chewing and swallowing

FIGURE 7. Universal sign of choking (hands clutching the throat).

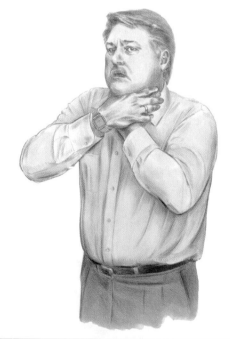

Foundation Facts: Causes of Airway Obstruction

There are 3 common causes of airway obstruction in adults. Each is treated differently.

1. **Foreign body:** A foreign body (for example, food) may become lodged in the air passage and block the airway. If an adult has signs of severe or complete FBAO, give abdominal thrusts (the Heimlich maneuver) until the object is expelled or the victim becomes unresponsive.

2. **Relaxed tongue:** In an unresponsive victim (for example, someone who has had a stroke, someone with a head injury, or someone in cardiac arrest), the tongue may fall back against the throat and block the airway. Use either the head tilt–chin lift or the jaw thrust (described in Chapter 2) to lift the tongue away from the back of the throat.

3. **Swollen air passages:** This condition is a *medical* problem that is caused by an infection or inflammation rather than a *mechanical* problem caused by a foreign body. Medications are needed to treat swollen air passages, and the victim may require assistance with breathing. Abdominal thrusts or other CPR techniques will *not* relieve this type of airway obstruction. Airway obstruction that is caused by swollen air passages typically develops gradually with other signs of respiratory failure or distress, such as a gradual increase in wheezing in a person with asthma. In contrast, airway obstruction caused by a foreign body typically develops suddenly and causes *sudden* coughing and *sudden* difficulty breathing.

Protecting Your Heart and Blood Vessels

The blood vessels in your heart and brain require special care to remain healthy and clear of obstructions. Cigarette smoking, high blood pressure, a diet high in fat, and other factors can damage blood vessels and obstruct blood flow. If your blood vessels are damaged or obstructed, they will gradually narrow. Blood clots will form, resulting in a heart attack or stroke.

The Table lists the major controllable risk factors of heart attack and stroke. Review these risk factors and the lifestyle changes needed to reduce your risk of heart attack and stroke.

Other risk factors for heart attack and stroke are heredity, male gender, increasing age, diabetes, stress, and race (African Americans have the greatest risk of heart attack and stroke). The following short quiz can help you identify risk factors for heart attack. To learn more about preventing heart attack and stroke, contact your local AHA or visit the AHA website at www.americanheart.org.

TABLE. Major Controllable Risk Factors of Heart Attack and Stroke

Factor	Explanation	Lifestyle Behavior to Reduce Risk
Cigarette smoking	Cigarette smoking is the leading preventable cause of death in the United States. Smoking and second-hand smoke can damage blood vessels and cause many other preventable diseases. Secondhand smoke hurts your loved ones.	Stop smoking as soon as possible. Pick a day *now* to quit. Ask your doctor for help. The greatest gift you can give yourself, your loved ones, and your friends is to quit smoking.
High blood pressure	High blood pressure increases the risk of heart attack and stroke. High blood pressure can damage blood vessels, including those in the brain.	Have your blood pressure checked at least once a year and more often if it is elevated. If you have high blood pressure, see a physician and take your medications as instructed.
High blood cholesterol	Excess cholesterol can be deposited on the inner walls of the arteries, narrowing them. This will reduce blood flow to the heart or brain.	Have your blood cholesterol levels checked regularly. Avoid a diet high in saturated fat.
Lack of exercise	Lack of exercise contributes to factors that cause a heart attack. But vigorous exercise by people who have not exercised regularly can be dangerous. Consult a physician before starting an exercise program.	With your physician's help, plan a program for regular exercise and stick to it.
Obesity	Obesity increases the risk of high blood pressure, diabetes, and high blood cholesterol. All of these conditions increase the risk of heart attack and stroke.	Develop a healthy diet with help from your physician. Fad diets do not produce long-term weight loss.
Heart disease	Heart disease is a major risk factor for heart attack and stroke.	Follow your doctor's advice for treating heart disease.
Transient ischemic attacks (TIAs)	TIAs are strokelike symptoms that disappear in less than 24 hours. TIAs are strong predictors of stroke. If they are detected and the patient is treated, it may be possible to reduce the risk of subsequent stroke. They are usually treated with drugs that keep blood clots from forming.	If strokelike symptoms occur, phone 911 or other emergency response number and seek immediate evaluation in the nearest Emergency Department.

Are You at Risk for a Heart Attack?

The following factors increase the risk of heart attack. Check all that apply to you. If you have 2 or more risk factors, see a physician for a complete evaluation of your risk.

Men

❏ Are you more than 45 years old?

Women

❏ Are you more than 55 years old?

❏ Are you past menopause?

❏ Have your ovaries been removed and if so, you're not taking estrogen?

Both

❏ Did your father or brother have a heart attack before age 55?

❏ Did your mother or sister have a heart attack before age 65?

❏ Did your mother, father, sister, brother, or grandparent have a stroke?

❏ Do you smoke or live or work with others who smoke tobacco daily?

❏ Is your total cholesterol level 240 mg/dL or higher?

❏ You don't know your total cholesterol level?

❏ Is your high-density lipoprotein (HDL) ("good") cholesterol less than 35 mg/dL?

❏ You don't know your HDL level?

❏ Is your blood pressure 140/90 mm Hg or higher?

❏ Have you been told that your blood pressure is too high?

❏ You don't know your blood pressure?

❏ Do you exercise for less than 30 minutes on most days?

❏ Are you 20 pounds or more overweight for your height and build?

❏ Is your fasting blood sugar level 128 mg/dL or higher?

❏ Do you need medicine to control your blood sugar level?

❏ Do you have coronary artery disease?

❏ Have you had a heart attack?

❏ Have you had a stroke or transient ischemic attack?

To learn more about preventing heart attack and stroke, phone your local American Heart Association (1-800-242-8721) or visit the AHA Web site at www.americanheart.org.

Summary

To rescue someone with a cardiovascular emergency, you must first recognize that the person is having an emergency. The Chain of Survival for heart attack, cardiac arrest, stroke, and FBAO starts with YOU, someone who is trained to recognize the emergency and take action. Recognizing warning signs is an important step that you will practice again and again in this course.

We encourage you to become a part of the community's Chain of Survival. Healthcare providers are an important part of the community Chain of Survival and the Chain of Survival in any medical facility. In this course you will learn to

- Recognize the signs of heart attack, cardiac arrest, stroke, and FBAO (choking) in adults
- Phone 911 or other emergency response number in your area for these emergencies
- Perform CPR and use an AED

With this knowledge and these skills, you will become an effective and vital link in the Chain of Survival.

Learning Checklist

Review the key information you learned in this chapter.

- The 4 links in the AHA Adult Chain of Survival are
  - Early access to the emergency response system
  - Early CPR
  - Early defibrillation
  - Early advanced care
- Early defibrillation is needed to treat VF. The sooner defibrillation is attempted, the better the victim's chance of survival.
- AEDs are operated by trained healthcare providers and lay rescuers. Providing defibrillation within the first few minutes after collapse greatly improves the victim's chance of survival.

- Signs and symptoms of heart attack:
  - The most common symptom of a heart attack is a pain, pressure, squeezing, or heaviness in the center of the chest behind the breastbone (sternum). The pain may travel to the neck, jaw, or arm (usually the left arm).
  - Many people (particularly women, people with diabetes, and the elderly) have vague signs and symptoms of a heart attack, such as sweaty skin, lightheadedness, fainting, shortness of breath, nausea, and discomfort described as an ache, heartburn, or indigestion.
- The 3 *red flags* of cardiac arrest are
  - No response
  - No normal breathing
  - No signs of circulation (normal breathing, coughing, or movement)
- The 3 *red flags* of stroke are the sudden development of
  - Facial droop
  - Arm weakness
  - Speech difficulties
- The 6 *red flags* of severe or complete FBAO (choking) are
  - Universal sign of choking (hands clutching the throat)
  - Inability to speak (ask "Can you speak?")
  - Weak, ineffective, or silent coughs
  - High-pitched sounds while inhaling
  - Increased difficulty breathing
  - Blue lips and skin (cyanosis)

Review Questions

1. You enter a patient's room. You discover your 64-year-old female patient lying unresponsive on the floor. What do you do?

   a. shout for help — if no one responds, leave the patient to phone the emergency response number.

   b. shout for help and begin CPR

   c. perform rescue breathing until help arrives

   d. transfer the patient to advanced care

2. During a visit to the clinic, a patient becomes pale and sweaty and complains of chest discomfort. You suspect he is having a heart attack. Which of the following is a *red flag* of heart attack that should prompt you to call the emergency response number?

   a. squeezing or crushing chest pain behind the breastbone that lasts more than a few minutes

   b. sharp, stabbing chest pain that lasts only a few seconds

   c. shortness of breath

   d. a headache the patient describes as "the worst headache of my life"

3. An elderly man in the registration area suddenly clutches his chest and collapses. You go to his aid and discover that he is unresponsive. You ask a bystander to phone the emergency response number. Which of the following signs or symptoms are the *red flags* of cardiac arrest?

   a. facial droop, arm weakness, and speech difficulties

   b. chest pain, lightheadedness, sweating, and nausea

   c. no response, no normal breathing, and no signs of circulation

   d. no response, spontaneous breathing, and chest pain

4. You are talking with your supervisor when she begins to slur her words. You suspect she is having a stroke. Which of the following signs or symptoms are the *red flags* of stroke that should prompt you to call the emergency response number?

   a. sudden loss of responsiveness and cardiac arrest

   b. sudden facial droop, arm weakness, and speech difficulties

   c. no response, no normal breathing, and no signs of circulation

   d. crushing chest pain that lasts a few minutes, nausea, and sweating

5. A 22-year-old woman at the table next to yours in the cafeteria suddenly begins coughing forcefully and then clutches her neck and becomes silent. Which of the following signs or symptoms are the *red flags* of severe or complete FBAO that prompt you to perform the Heimlich maneuver?

   a. wheezing between coughs and hoarse speech

   b. severe, forceful coughing

   c. inability to speak, breathe, or cough forcefully and blue skin or lips

   d. no response, no normal breathing, and no signs of circulation

How did you do?

Answers: **1,** a; **2,** a; **3,** c; **4,** b; **5,** c

You are working in a physicians' office building when Adam, a 55-year-old coworker, suddenly collapses. You shake his shoulder and shout at him, but he does not respond. You immediately tell another coworker to phone the medical center emergency response number (to activate the emergency response team) and get the AED. You open Adam's airway and look, listen, and feel for breathing. You detect no breaths. You quickly position the face shield that you carry with you and deliver 2 slow rescue breaths. You see his chest rise with each breath. You then check for signs of circulation (pulse, adequate breathing, coughing, and movement). You feel no pulse and you see no signs of any movement or breathing. You begin chest compressions at a rate of 100 compressions per minute, giving 2 rescue breaths after every 15 chest compressions.

Within 2 minutes coworkers arrive with emergency equipment, including a bag-mask system with supplemental oxygen and an AED. You continue chest compressions and rescue breathing until the AED electrode pads are ready to be attached. Then you stop compressions to allow attachment of the pads. Once the pads are attached, the AED analyzes Adam's heart rhythm and recommends a shock. You deliver that shock and the next 2 recommended shocks. After the third shock the AED indicates "no shock is advised, check the victim." You find that Adam is breathing adequately and has signs of circulation. The emergency response team arrives and transports Adam to the hospital.

A month later you attend Adam's "welcome back" party.*

*Modified from *BLS for Healthcare Providers,* Chapter 6: Adult Cardiopulmonary Resuscitation.

The ABCs of CPR: Adult CPR and Relief of FBAO

Overview

If you were involved in this case scenario, would you know what to do? In this chapter you will learn the steps of CPR. You begin the steps of CPR when you find an unresponsive adult.

CPR: The Second Link in the Adult Chain of Survival

CPR is the second link in the AHA adult Chain of Survival. CPR is a set of assessments and skills you perform to save the life of an unresponsive person. CPR maintains delivery of oxygen and blood to the heart and brain. The assessments and skills are performed in sequence so that you provide only the support the victim needs. CPR skills include a combination of rescue breathing (blowing) and chest compressions (pumping). You provide rescue breathing if the victim is not breathing and chest compressions if the victim has no signs of circulation.

CPR helps the victim even if ventricular fibrillation (VF) is present because CPR helps the heart respond better to defibrillation. You must begin CPR at once to provide oxygen to the heart and to increase the chance that defibrillation will succeed.

If you find an *unresponsive* person and other rescuers are nearby, send someone to phone 911 (or other emergency response number) and get the AED. *Then YOU start CPR.* Continue CPR until you can provide defibrillation or until other trained rescuers arrive. If you are alone, phone the emergency response number (or 911) and get the AED *first.* Then return to the victim to begin CPR.

Learning Objectives

After reading this chapter and practicing the skills you will be able to

1. Recognize cardiac arrest

2. Describe and demonstrate phoning the emergency response number, rescue breathing using the mouth-to-mouth and mouth-to–barrier device techniques, and rescue breathing using the bag-mask device

3. Describe and demonstrate the techniques of 1-rescuer and 2-rescuer CPR

4. Describe and demonstrate the technique of applying cricoid pressure while other rescuers provide bag-mask ventilation

5. Recognize the signs of foreign-body airway obstruction (choking)

6. Describe and demonstrate how to relieve foreign-body airway obstruction in both responsive and unresponsive adults

Note: The FYI box in Chapter 4, page 59, explains why a lone rescuer should "Phone First" for an unresponsive adult victim but "Phone Fast" after 1 minute of CPR for an unresponsive pediatric victim.

Critical Concepts:
Critical Actions to Take for an Unresponsive Adult

1. Dial 911 (or other emergency response number)

2. Get the AED

The Steps of CPR

The assessment and skills steps of CPR are called the ABCs of CPR. **A** stands for **airway, B** for **breathing,** and **C** for **circulation.** The assessment and skills steps are simple. At each step you assess the victim and then provide only the rescue support the victim needs (see Chapter 1, Figure 2).

1. **Check response. Check whether the victim is responsive** by gently shaking the victim and shouting "Are you OK?" (Figure 1A).

   ■ **If the victim is** *unresponsive,* **phone the emergency response number (or 911)** and get the AED (Figure 1B). Your call activates the emergency response system and ensures that help is on the way. The AHA recommends that AEDs be stored next to the telephone to ensure rapid access to both the emergency response number and the AED.

   ■ **If you are alone** and find an unresponsive adult, leave the victim to phone 911 or other emergency response number and get the AED.

   ■ If you or someone else has called the emergency response number, kneel at the victim's side near the head to start CPR. Carefully turn the victim onto the back if needed. If you think the victim is injured, turn the head, neck, and back as a unit.

FIGURE 1. A, Check for responsiveness by gently shaking the victim and shouting "Are you OK?" **B,** If a second rescuer is present, send that rescuer to phone 911 (or other emergency response number) and get the AED. You continue the steps of CPR.

A

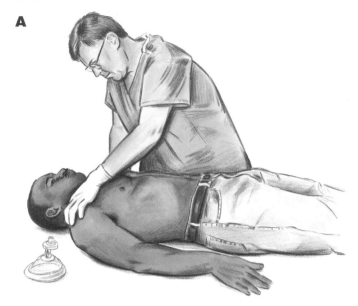

B

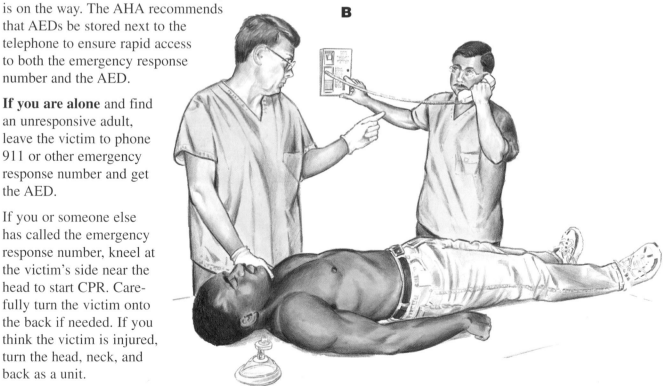

2. Airway: Open the airway. When a victim becomes unresponsive, the muscles of the jaw and neck relax. This allows the tongue to fall back against the throat and block the airway (Figure 2A). You must open the airway. There are 2 techniques for opening the airway:

FIGURE 2. Opening the airway with the head tilt–chin lift. **A,** In an unresponsive victim the tongue falls back and obstructs the airway. **B,** The head tilt–chin lift technique lifts the tongue away from the back of the throat and opens the airway.

A

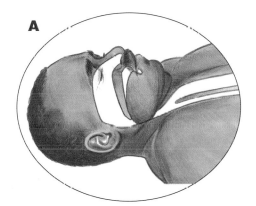

B

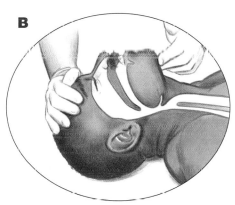

FIGURE 3. Opening the airway with the jaw thrust. Lifting the angles of the jaw moves the jaw and tongue forward and opens the airway without bending the neck. Use the jaw thrust when you think the victim has a head or neck injury.

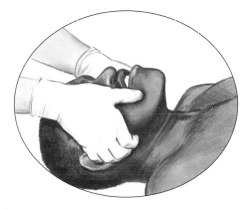

- *Head tilt–chin lift:* Place the palm of one hand on the victim's forehead and apply firm, backward pressure, tilting the head back. Gently lift the chin with the other hand (Figure 2B). This lifts the tongue away from the back of the throat.

- *Jaw thrust:* If you think the victim's head or neck is injured, use the *jaw thrust* (Figure 3) to open the airway. Lift the angles of the jaw (the part of the jaw right below the earlobes). This moves the jaw and tongue forward and opens the airway without bending the neck.

FYI: Opening the Airway

In CPR your first action is to open the airway. In an unresponsive victim the muscles of the jaw and neck relax. This allows the tongue to fall back against the throat and block the airway (Figure 2A). The tongue is the most common cause of a blocked airway in an unresponsive victim.

There are 2 techniques to pull the tongue away from the back of the throat and open the airway: the head tilt–chin lift and the jaw thrust. Both techniques lift the jaw because the tongue is attached to the lower jaw. When you lift the jaw you also lift the tongue away from the back of the throat.

Head tilt–chin lift: To perform the head tilt–chin lift, use the palm of one hand to apply firm, backward pressure to the victim's forehead. This will tilt the head back. Place the fingers of the other hand under the bony part of the lower jaw near the chin. Lift the jaw upward to bring the chin forward. This will lift the tongue away from the back of the throat and open the airway.

The head tilt–chin lift is the most frequently used method of opening the airway, so this method is emphasized in this course. If the victim has a head or neck injury, you must prevent any movement of the head or neck. To open the airway in injured victims, use the jaw thrust.

Jaw thrust: If you think the victim has a head or neck injury, use only the *jaw thrust* to open the airway (Figure 4). *Do not use the head tilt–chin lift in victims with a head or neck injury. The head tilt–chin lift may worsen the injury in these victims.*

To perform the jaw thrust, place your fingers under the angles of the victim's jaw (the part of the jaw right below the earlobes). Lift the jaw *without* tilting the head. The jaw thrust will pull the tongue away from the back of the throat without moving the head or neck. Use the jaw thrust to open the airway when you think the victim has an injury to the head or neck.

3. **Breathing.** Hold the airway open and *look, listen, and feel* to determine if the victim is breathing adequately (Figure 4). If the victim is not breathing adequately, give 2 slow rescue breaths.

To check for breathing, look, listen, and feel for breathing:

a. Place your ear next to the victim's mouth and nose and turn your head to look at the chest.

b. Look for the chest to rise, listen for sounds of normal breathing, and feel for air movement on your cheek.

If the victim is not breathing adequately, give rescue breaths. Healthcare providers can give rescue breaths in 3 ways:

■ Mouth-to-mouth or mouth-to-nose technique

■ Mouth-to–barrier device technique

■ Bag-mask technique

This section addresses rescue breathing with the mouth-to-mouth and mouth-to-nose techniques (Figure 5A and 5B). Rescue breathing with barrier and bag-mask devices is presented in the next section.

To use the mouth-to mouth or mouth-to-nose technique:

a. Place your mouth around the victim's mouth and pinch the nose closed (Figure 5A), or close the victim's mouth and place your mouth around the victim's nose (Figure 5B).

FIGURE 4. Place your ear next to the victim's mouth and nose and look at the victim's chest. *Look* for the chest to rise, *listen* for sounds of breathing, and *feel* for breath on your cheek.

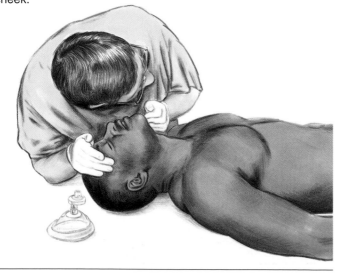

FIGURE 5. Rescue breathing. **A,** Mouth-to-mouth technique. **B,** Mouth-to-nose technique.

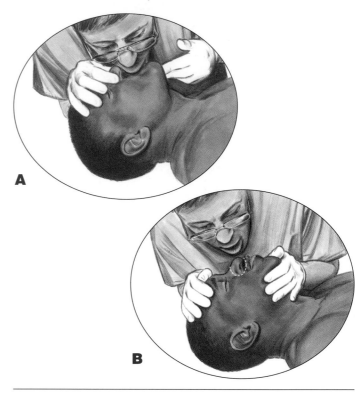

A

B

---

b. Continue to tilt the head and lift the chin (or perform the jaw thrust).

c. Give 2 slow breaths (about 2 seconds each). Deliver breaths *slowly.* If you deliver breaths too quickly or too forcefully, you will force air into the stomach instead of the lungs.

d. *Be sure the victim's chest rises each time you give a rescue breath. If the chest does not rise, reopen the airway and give rescue breaths again.*

e. Healthcare providers must be able to provide rescue breathing with the mouth-to-mouth or mouth-to-nose technique, with a barrier device (face shield or face mask), and with a bag-mask device. Use of those devices and more details on rescue breathing are described later in this chapter. You are providing adequate ventilation if you see the chest rise and fall with each breath and you hear and feel the air escaping during exhalation.

■ When you give rescue breaths *without supplemental oxygen,* give them for 2 seconds. The chest rise should clearly rise with each breath.

■ When you give rescue breaths through a mask barrier device or a bag-mask device *with supplemental oxygen,* you can use a smaller volume for each breath. Smaller breaths can be used because the air is enriched with oxygen, so smaller breaths will still help supply oxygen to the blood. *Deliver these smaller breaths over 1 to 2 seconds.* These smaller breaths should still make the chest rise, but the rise does not need to be as pronounced as when you are delivering breaths without oxygen (see below).

Foundation Facts:
Why Is Rescue Breathing Important?

When breathing stops, delivery of oxygen to the heart and brain stops. If delivery of oxygen is not restored quickly, the heart and brain will be damaged. The longer the victim is deprived of oxygen, the smaller the chance that he or she will survive. Even if chest compressions are effective or defibrillation restores a normal heart rhythm, it may take several minutes for a victim to begin breathing adequately again. Mouth-to-mouth breathing is the quickest way to deliver oxygen to the victim's lungs and blood.

When you give rescue breaths, be sure the victim's chest rises with each breath. The chest should rise with each breath whether you give the breaths with mouth-to-mouth, mouth-to-mask, or bag-mask ventilation. It is critical to look for the chest to rise because chest rise is the sign that you are giving effective rescue breaths. *If the chest does not rise when you give breaths, reopen the airway and give rescue breaths again.*

Deliver rescue breaths *slowly.* Take 2 seconds to deliver each breath. Do not give rapid, forceful breaths. Such breaths will blow air into the esophagus and stomach instead of the lungs. Air in the stomach can cause vomiting, which makes CPR more difficult.

If a victim has dentures, leave them in place unless they are extremely loose. Dentures help provide a good mouth-to-mouth seal. If the dentures are loose, remove them. Loose dentures will not help you make a good mouth-to-mouth seal, and they may fall back into the throat and block the airway.

4. **Circulation.** After you give 2 rescue breaths, look for signs of circulation:

   a. Look for adequate breathing, coughing, or movement in response to the 2 rescue breaths, and try to feel a carotid pulse (see Critical Concepts: Checking for Signs of Circulation). To check the carotid pulse, locate the victim's windpipe (trachea) with your index and middle fingers (Figure 6A) and slide your fingers in the groove between the windpipe and the muscle at the side of the neck (Figure 6B).

   b. Do not take more than 10 seconds to check for signs of circulation.

   c. If you do not confidently feel a pulse or see other signs of circulation, start chest compressions and be prepared to use an AED.

   Note: If the victim has signs of circulation, chest compressions are *not* required and you should *not* attach AED electrode pads. If the victim is not breathing adequately but has signs of circulation, the victim is in respiratory arrest, and you must continue to give rescue breaths (1 breath every 5 seconds).

FIGURE 6. Checking the carotid pulse. **A,** Locate the windpipe (also called the trachea). **B,** Slide your fingers into the groove between the windpipe and the muscle at the side of the neck.

A

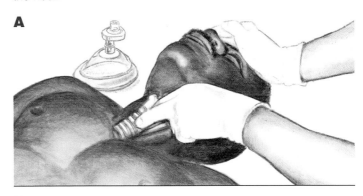

B

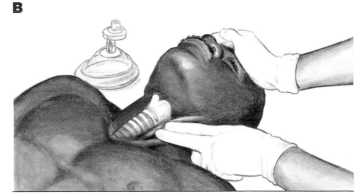

Critical Concepts:
Checking for Signs of Circulation

Blood must circulate to deliver oxygen to the brain, heart, and other vital organs. If you can feel a pulse or if you identify signs of adequate breathing, coughing, or movement in response to the 2 rescue breaths, signs of circulation are present. If signs of circulation are present, chest compressions and defibrillation are unnecessary. If you are unsure whether you feel a pulse or see signs of circulation, begin chest compressions.

The AHA recommends that both lay rescuers and healthcare providers look for signs of circulation. When *lay rescuers* check for signs of circulation, they look for *normal* breathing, coughing, and movement in response to the 2 rescue breaths. When *healthcare providers* check for signs of circulation, they check for a *carotid pulse* and *adequate* breathing, coughing, and movement in response to the rescue breaths. As a healthcare provider you must be able to judge if breathing is adequate to support oxygenation. To do this you must distinguish between adequate and inadequate breathing (such as agonal breathing).

d. Chest compressions are performed on the *lower half* of the sternum (breastbone). To locate the correct position for chest compressions,

■ Place your fingers on the lower margin of the victim's rib cage on the side nearest you (Figure 7A).

■ Slide your fingers up the rib cage to the notch where the ribs meet the lower sternum (in the center of the lower part of the chest).

■ Place the heel of one hand on the lower half of the sternum and the other hand on top of the first so that the hands are parallel (Figure 7B).

■ Locate the compression point on the breastbone by finding the part of the breastbone between the victim's nipples (Figures 7C and 8).

■ Lean forward so your shoulders are over the breastbone and your arms are straight (Figure 8). You should be looking down at your hands.

■ You may extend or interlace your fingers, but do not rest them on the chest. Keep the heel of your hand on the chest during and between compressions.

e. Provide 15 compressions at a rate of about 100 compressions per minute.

Note: The rate of compressions is slightly fewer than 2 compressions per second. You will actually deliver fewer than 100 compressions per minute because you will stop compressions to give rescue breaths (see FYI: Difference Between Compression *Rate* and the Number of Compressions Actually *Delivered* per Minute).

■ Compress (push down on) the breastbone 1½ to 2 inches with each compression.

■ Allow the chest to relax (come back to its normal shape) between compressions, but leave the heel of your hand on the chest between compressions. Do not lift your hands off the chest.

If you have difficulty compressing the chest 1½ to 2 inches, try a different hand position. Grasp the wrist of the hand on the chest with your other hand and push downward with both. This technique is helpful for rescuers with arthritis.

Provide 15 compressions, and then give 2 rescue breaths.

FIGURE 7. Chest compressions. **A,** Identify the lower margin of the ribs and the lowest part of the breastbone (or sternum). **B,** Compress the lower half of the breastbone, being careful to avoid the very bottom of the breastbone. **C,** The proper location for chest compressions is between the nipples. This position corresponds to the lower half of the sternum.

A

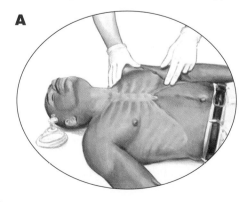

B

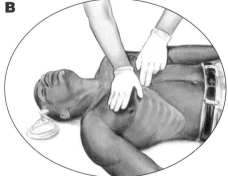

C

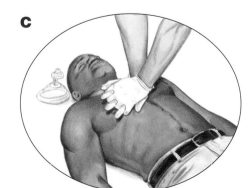

FIGURE 8. Proper hand position and position of the rescuer to perform chest compressions.

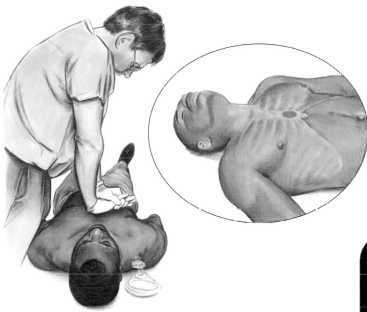

5. **Continue to provide cycles of 15 chest compressions and 2 rescue breaths.** After 1 minute of CPR (about 4 cycles of 15 compressions and 2 breaths), check for signs of circulation, including a pulse. If signs of circulation return, stop chest compressions and continue providing rescue breathing if needed (1 breath every 5 seconds). If you do not detect signs of circulation, continue cycles of 15 chest compressions and 2 breaths until an AED or ALS rescuers arrive. Check for signs of circulation every few minutes.

FYI: Difference Between Compression *Rate* and the Number of Compressions Actually *Delivered* per Minute

During adult CPR you compress the sternum at *a rate of 100 times per minute*. This corresponds to a rate slightly less than 2 compressions per second during each set of 15 compressions, so it won't take too many seconds to perform each set of compressions. The term *compression rate* refers to the *speed* of compressions, not the actual *number* of compressions delivered per minute.

The recommended compression rate will actually provide less than 100 compressions each minute because you will pause to provide breaths after every 15 compressions. The actual number of compressions delivered per minute will vary from rescuer to rescuer. The number of compressions is influenced not only by the compression rate but also by the speed with which you position the head, open the airway, and deliver rescue breaths.

The *rate* of chest compressions can be likened to the speed you drive in a car. If you drive 100 miles per hour but stop briefly every 15 miles, at the end of 1 hour you will have driven less than 100 miles.

Foundation Facts: Agonal Breathing and Respiratory Arrest

Victims of cardiac arrest soon stop breathing. Some victims may have irregular, infrequent, gasping, or shallow breaths. These breaths are called "agonal breaths." Agonal breaths do not provide enough oxygen for the victim. Agonal breaths may fool some rescuers into thinking that the victim is still breathing and does not need rescue breathing or other steps of CPR. If you do not provide rescue breathing, you might miss an opportunity to save a person's life.

If the victim is unresponsive and is not breathing *adequately,* give 2 rescue breaths and be sure the chest rises with each breath. Then check for signs of circulation, including a pulse. If the victim has no signs of circulation (no pulse and no adequate breathing, no coughing, and no movement in response to the 2 rescue breaths), the victim is in cardiac arrest.

A victim in *respiratory arrest* is unresponsive and is not breathing adequately but does have signs of circulation (for example, a pulse). This victim requires rescue breathing but does not need chest compressions or defibrillation. Do *not* attach AED electrode pads to victims in respiratory arrest.

A victim in *cardiac arrest* is unresponsive, is not breathing adequately, and has no signs of circulation (including no pulse). This victim requires all the steps of CPR (compressions and rescue breaths) and defibrillation.

CPR Performed by 2 Rescuers

All professional rescuers (BLS ambulance providers, healthcare professionals, and laypersons who have a duty to perform, such as lifeguards or police) should learn both 1-rescuer and 2-rescuer techniques. When you perform CPR in the workplace, particularly in a healthcare facility, use barrier devices such as mouth-to-mask devices or bag-mask ventilation.

In 2-rescuer CPR, 1 rescuer is positioned at the victim's side and performs chest compressions. The other rescuer remains at the victim's head, keeps the airway open, monitors the carotid pulse (if the rescuer is a healthcare provider) to assess the effectiveness of chest compressions, and provides rescue breathing (Figure 9).

FIGURE 9. Two-rescuer CPR. One rescuer is positioned at the victim's head to open the airway, perform rescue breathing, monitor the effectiveness of chest compressions, and check for signs of circulation. The second rescuer is positioned at the-victim's side to provide chest compressions.

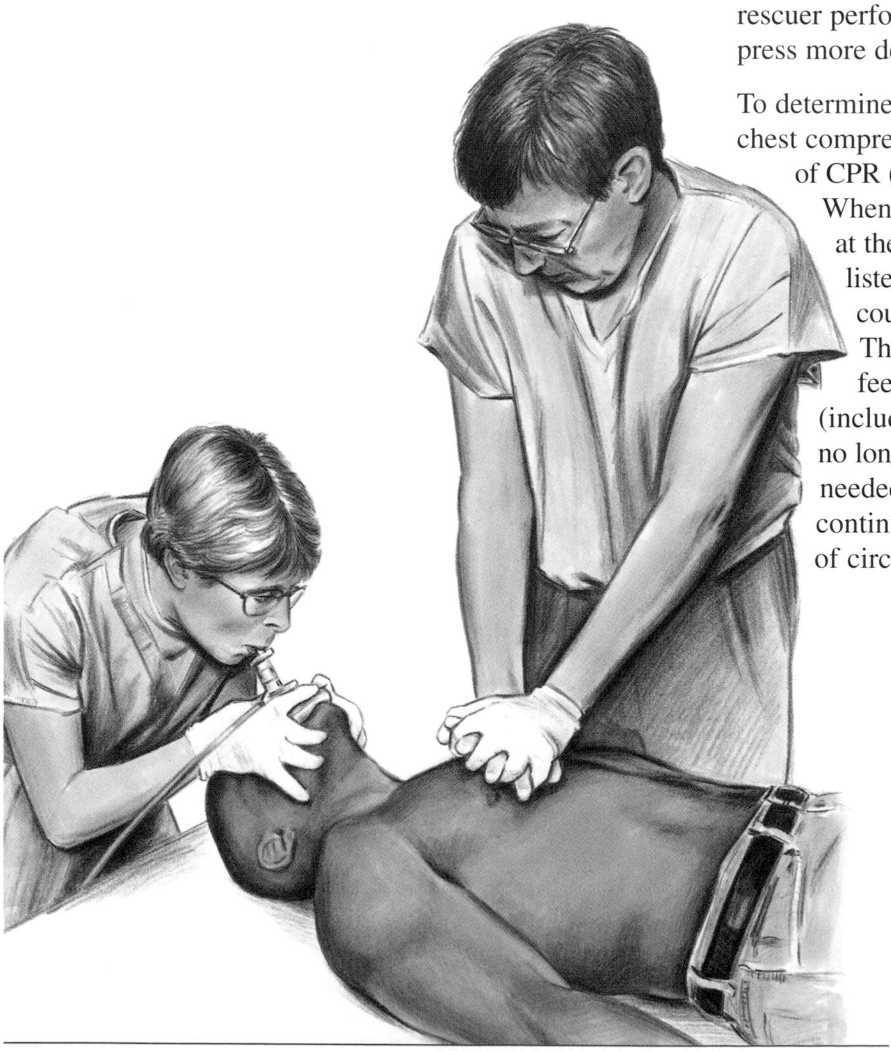

The compression rate for 2-rescuer CPR is 100 compressions per minute. The compression-ventilation ratio for 2-rescuer adult CPR is 15:2. This ratio is the number of compressions (15) and breaths (2) in 1 cycle. Provide cycles of 15 compressions and 2 breaths until a breathing (tracheal) tube is inserted. Take 2 seconds for each rescue breath. The victim exhales between the 2 breaths and during the first chest compression immediately after the second breath. Once a breathing tube is inserted, the compression-ventilation ratio is asynchronous (compression rate of about 100/minute, ventilation rate of 12 to 15 breaths per minute).

Performing chest compressions is tiring. If 1 rescuer becomes tired, change positions. Change quickly. Interrupting chest compressions interrupts circulation.

Reassessment During 2-Rescuer CPR

During 2-rescuer CPR the rescuer giving breaths must assess the effectiveness of chest compressions and must periodically check for signs of circulation. To assess the effectiveness of chest compressions, feel for a pulse during chest compressions. If you do not feel a pulse, the rescuer performing chest compressions will need to compress more deeply or forcefully.

To determine if the victim has signs of circulation, stop chest compressions for 10 seconds after the first minute of CPR (or according to the protocol at your facility). When chest compressions are stopped, the rescuer at the victim's head opens the airway and looks, listens, and feels for adequate breathing or coughing. Both rescuers look for movement. The rescuer at the victim's head should also feel for a carotid pulse. If signs of circulation (including a pulse) return, chest compressions are no longer required. Rescue breathing may still be needed. If no signs of circulation are detected, continue chest compressions and check for signs of circulation every few minutes.

Recovery Position

If signs of circulation return, chest compressions are unnecessary. Continue rescue breathing until the victim breathes adequately. If the victim starts to breathe adequately and no signs of injury are present, place the victim in the recovery position (see Figure 10 and Foundation Facts: The Recovery Position). If the victim is injured, leave the victim on his back and hold the airway open using a jaw thrust as needed.

FIGURE 10. Recovery positions. There are several recovery positions. Place the victim in a position that supports the head and neck in a neutral position. Make sure there is no pressure on joints and bony prominences.

Foundation Facts:
The Recovery Position

If the victim is unresponsive but breathing adequately, neither cardiac nor respiratory arrest is present. Such a victim does not need chest compressions or rescue breathing. If there are no signs of injury, place the victim in a recovery position (Figure 10). A recovery position keeps the airway open.

To place the victim in a recovery position, kneel beside the victim and straighten the victim's legs. Roll the victim toward you onto his or her side. Position the top leg to balance the victim on his or her side. Tilt the victim's head to a neutral position to keep the airway open.

Continue to check the victim. Frequently check breathing (look, listen, and feel). If the victim stops breathing, turn the victim onto his or her back, phone 911 (or other emergency response number) and get the AED (or be sure someone else does), and begin CPR.

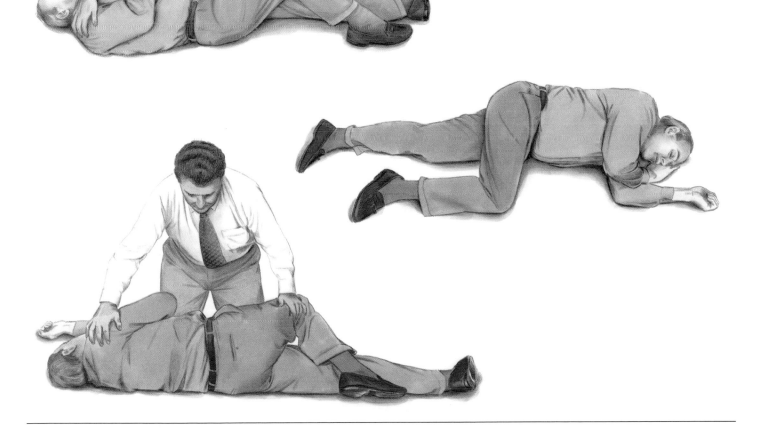

Face Shields, Mouth-to-Mask Devices, and Bag-Mask Devices

Mouth-to-mouth rescue breathing may be lifesaving for victims and is safe for rescuers. When you perform CPR you have almost no chance of becoming infected with viruses such as human immunodeficiency virus (HIV), the virus that causes AIDS, or any hepatitis virus. No human has ever contracted HIV or hepatitis through mouth-to-mouth contact during CPR.

Nonetheless the AHA recommends that healthcare providers use barrier devices or bag-mask devices to provide rescue breathing in the workplace. The Occupational Safety and Health Administration (OSHA) requires that "universal precautions" be followed when there is any exposure to blood or bodily fluids, including saliva. Universal precautions include the use of barrier devices during rescue breathing. Employees expected to perform CPR in the workplace (for example, healthcare providers) should use barrier devices.

Use bag-mask devices with supplemental oxygen to provide rescue breathing whenever possible. Equipment to support ventilation — pocket masks or bag-mask devices — should be readily available in all patient care rooms and all patient care areas. They should also be placed on the resuscitation cart. Remember, though, a barrier device is *not* required to perform CPR. That is why this manual provides instruction about mouth-to-mouth and mouth-to-nose rescue breathing.

Regardless of whether a barrier device is available, the key actions of the rescuer are the same:

1. Open the airway using the head tilt–chin lift (or jaw thrust if the victim has head or neck injuries)

2. Provide rescue breaths lasting 2 seconds each. If you are using a barrier device, position the face shield or face mask over the victim's mouth and ensure an adequate air seal. Give rescue breaths through the barrier device. Use enough force to make the chest rise with each breath.

There are 2 types of barrier devices, face shields and face masks. In this course you will learn how to use the barrier device available in your workplace and a bag-mask device. Correct use of these devices requires practice. Practice rescue breathing with these devices on a manikin several times. The most critical step in using a face shield, face mask, or bag-mask device is creation of a good seal around the mouth and nose. A good seal prevents leakage of air during rescue breaths.

Face Shields

Face shields are clear plastic or silicon sheets. You place the shield over the victim's face to keep your mouth from directly touching the victim's mouth. All face shields have an opening or tube in the center of the sheet. You will give rescue breaths through this opening. Face shields are small, flexible, and portable. A folded shield will fit easily in a packet on a key ring. If you keep the packet on your key ring, it is likely to be available when you need it.

Using a Face Shield

To use a face shield (Figure 11) during rescue breathing:

- Unwrap and unfold the face shield.

- Place the face shield with the opening or tube over the victim's mouth. Make sure the plastic covers the victim's nose.

- Perform the head tilt–chin lift to open the airway.

- Pinch the victim's nose closed and place your mouth over the opening or tube.

- Give 2 slow rescue breaths (take 2 seconds for each) and watch the chest to see if it rises. The victim's exhaled air will escape between the shield and his or her face when you lift your mouth off the shield.

Leave the face shield on the victim's face between rescue breaths (while chest compressions are performed). Replace the face shield with a mouth-to-mask barrier device or a bag-mask device with supplemental oxygen as soon as either is available.

FIGURE 11. Rescuer preparing to perform rescue breathing with a face shield in place. During rescue breathing the rescuer must ensure that the chest rises with each breath.

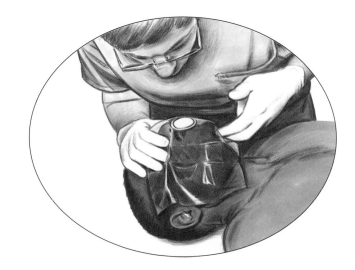

Face Masks

Face masks (Figure 12) are made of firm plastic with a cushioned rim. The rim creates a flexible seal around the victim's nose and mouth. Face masks are triangular in shape. The mask fits over the victim's mouth and nose. The narrowest portion of the mask is placed over the bridge of the victim's nose. Face masks are much easier to use than face shields. But they are bulkier, they cost more, and they are inconvenient to carry. This makes them less likely to be available if you unexpectedly have to perform CPR. Nonetheless face masks are the most common type of barrier device used in healthcare facilities. Most face masks have a 1-way valve that prevents exchange of bacteria or viruses between the victim and rescuer. Some masks have an oxygen inlet that permits administration of supplemental oxygen during rescue breathing.

Using a Face Mask

Most face masks are stored in a plastic container or bag. Some masks require assembly before they can be used. Become familiar with the face mask you expect to use *before* you need to use it. Make sure you can assemble the mask within seconds.

Rescuers who use a face mask kneel beside the victim (lateral technique) or at the top of the victim's head (cephalic technique).

FIGURE 12. Face mask. This barrier device is used to provide rescue breathing. Most face masks can be connected to an oxygen source. This allows delivery of supplemental oxygen during rescue breathing.

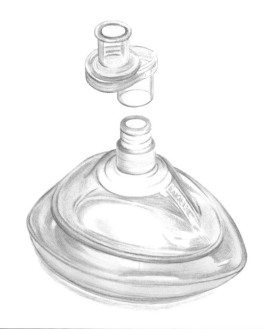

Lateral Technique

The lateral technique is the most convenient technique for 1-rescuer CPR. To use the face mask, kneel beside the victim in a location that will allow you to perform both rescue breathing and chest compressions. Then do the following (Figure 13A):

- Apply the mask to the victim's face. Use the bridge of the nose as a guide for correct positioning.

- Use the hand that is closer to the top of the victim's head to seal the mask to the victim's face. Place the index finger and thumb of that hand along the edge of the mask.

- Place the thumb of your other hand (the hand closer to the victim's feet) along the lower edge of the mask. Place the remaining fingers of that hand along the bony part of the jaw and lift the jaw using a head tilt–chin lift.

- Compress the mask firmly to create a tight seal between the mask and the victim's face.

- Give 2 slow rescue breaths. Be sure the chest rises with each breath.

Cephalic Technique

Use the cephalic technique for 2-rescuer CPR or for 1-rescuer CPR when only rescue breathing is needed. To provide rescue breathing using the cephalic technique, kneel directly above the victim's head and do the following (Figure 13B):

- Apply the mask to the victim's face. Use the bridge of the nose as a guide for correct positioning.

- Place your thumbs and the base of each thumb along the sides of the mask.

- Place both index fingers behind the angles of the jaw. Lift the jaw into the mask as you tilt the head back.

- While lifting the jaw, squeeze the mask against the victim's face with your thumbs and the heels of your hands. Squeeze firmly to achieve an airtight seal.

- Provide slow rescue breaths (2 seconds). Be sure the chest rises with each breath.

Another way to hold the mask in place is the E-C technique. Using the thumb and index finger of each hand to make a "C," press around the edges of the mask. Use the remaining fingers to lift the angles of the jaw (3 fingers form an "E") and open the airway (Figure 13C).

With either variation of the cephalic technique, you will use both hands to hold the mask and open the airway. In victims you think have a head or neck injury, lift the angles of the jaw but *do not* tilt the head to open the airway.

FIGURE 13. Use of a face mask. **A,** Lateral technique. This technique is most convenient for the lone rescuer who must also perform chest compressions. **B,** Cephalic technique. The face mask is held in place with the thumb and the side of each hand. **C,** Alternative cephalic E-C technique. The thumb and index finger of each hand form a "C" to hold the mask. The remaining 3 fingers of each hand (forming an "E") lift the jaw and keep the airway open. The cephalic technique is used for 2-rescuer CPR. In all 3 techniques the rescuer who gives breaths holds the mask firmly against the face and keeps the airway open.

A

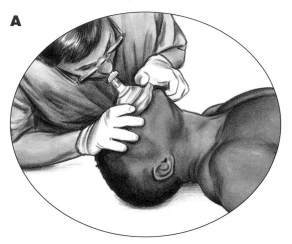

B

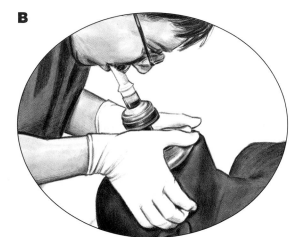

C

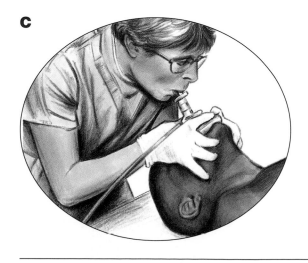

Effective use of the face mask requires instruction and supervised practice. During 2-rescuer CPR the mask can be used in a variety of ways. The most appropriate method will depend on the experience of personnel and the equipment available. Oral airways and cricoid pressure may be used with mouth-to-mask and any other form of rescue breathing.

If oxygen is unavailable, rescue breaths for mouth-to-mask breathing should be approximately the same volume as the volume used for mouth-to-mouth breathing (in adults deliver breaths over 2 seconds). Be sure each rescue breath makes the chest rise clearly.

If supplemental oxygen (minimum flow, 10 L/min, providing an inspired oxygen concentration of 40% or more) is available and joined to the mask during mouth-to-mask breathing, the rescuer can deliver smaller rescue breaths to the victim because the breaths are rich in oxygen. Deliver smaller breaths over 1 to 2 seconds. Be sure the chest rises with each breath, but remember that the rise does not need to be substantial when supplemental oxygen is used. If the victim is in respiratory arrest, you can assess the effectiveness of mouth-to-mask breathing with supplemental oxygen by monitoring the victim's oxygen saturation.

Bag-Mask Devices

Bag-mask devices consist of a self-inflating bag and a nonrebreathing valve attached to a face mask. The non-rebreathing valve directs exhaled air from the victim into the environment so that the victim does not rebreathe exhaled air. These devices are the most commonly used method of delivering rescue breaths by EMS providers and in hospitals. Most bag-mask units have adequate volume to provide effective rescue breaths and make the chest rise. A lone rescuer may have difficulty obtaining an airtight seal to the face while squeezing the bag and maintaining an open airway. For this reason bag-mask devices are most effective when 2 trained and experienced rescuers work together. One rescuer seals the mask to the face, and the other squeezes the bag slowly for 2 seconds (see below).

When you use a face mask or bag-mask *with* supplemental oxygen, you can give smaller rescue breaths (about 500 mL delivered over 1 to 2 seconds) than when you give rescue breaths *without* supplemental oxygen. Use of smaller breaths reduces the chance of air entering the stomach, vomiting, and aspiration (breathing in fluid or other foreign matter into the lungs). But smaller breaths should be used only if supplemental oxygen is delivered to the victim during rescue breathing through a mask (minimum oxygen flow rate of 10 L/min for the face mask and

8 to 12 L/min for the bag mask). When you use a bag-mask device *with* oxygen, squeeze the bag slowly for 1 to 2 seconds until the chest rises.

Using a Bag-Mask Device

Providing rescue breaths with a bag-mask device requires instruction and practice. The rescuer must be able to use the equipment effectively in a variety of situations.

If you are the only rescuer available for respiratory support you can use the E-C technique:

- Position yourself at the top of the victim's head (Figure 14).

- If there is no concern about neck injury, tilt the victim's head back and place it on a towel or pillow. If the victim has a head or neck injury, use a jaw thrust to open the airway. Do not move the head or neck.

- Apply the mask to the victim's face with one hand. Use the bridge of the nose as a guide for correct positioning.

- Place the thumb and index finger of that hand around the top of the mask (forming a "C"), and use the third, fourth, and fifth fingers of that hand (forming an "E") to lift the jaw and hold the airway open.

- Maintain head tilt and seal the mask firmly against the face.

- Compress the bag with your other hand. Watch the chest to be sure it rises.

- If supplemental oxygen is used, deliver each breath for 1 to 2 seconds. Be sure the chest rises with each breath. If room air is used, deliver slightly larger breaths for 2 seconds, making sure the chest clearly rises with each breath. Placing the bag next to your body may make it easier to compress the bag effectively. Maintain an airtight seal between the victim's face and the mask during delivery of each breath.

You may find the bag-mask device difficult to use effectively. Rescue breathing with a bag mask device is much easier when 2 rescuers use the bag-mask device as follows:

- One rescuer holds the mask to the victim's face and opens the victim's airway. The second rescuer squeezes the bag (Figure 15). To hold the mask to the victim's face, use the same techniques described for mouth-to-mask ventilation (the cephalic techniques).

- If a third rescuer is available and the victim is unconscious, the third rescuer can provide cricoid pressure (see the next page).

Bag-mask rescue breathing is a complex technique that requires considerable skill and practice. Practice using this device frequently.

FIGURE 14. Use of a bag-mask device by 1 rescuer. Circle the top edges of the mask with your thumb and index finger and lift the jaw with the remaining 3 fingers (E-C technique). Squeeze the bag while watching the chest to see if it rises. Creation of an airtight seal and maintenance of an open airway are the keys to successful use of the bag mask.

FIGURE 15. Use of the bag-mask device by 2 rescuers. The rescuer at the victim's head uses the E-C technique, with the thumb and index finger of each hand creating a "C" to provide a complete seal around the edges of the mask. This rescuer uses the remaining 3 fingers of each hand (the "E") to lift the victim's jaw and open the airway. The rescuer at the victim's side squeezes the bag and watches the chest to see if it rises.

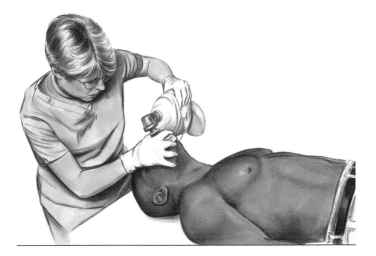

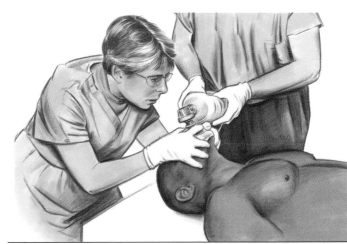

Cricoid Pressure (Sellick's Maneuver)

The cricoid pressure technique (Sellick's maneuver) applies pressure to the top of the unconscious victim's trachea (windpipe). This pushes the trachea backward, compressing the esophagus against the spinal column. During rescue breathing cricoid pressure prevents air from entering the esophagus and the stomach. This reduces the risk of vomiting and aspiration (entrance of stomach contents into the lungs). *Use cricoid pressure only if the victim is unconscious.*

Proper use of the cricoid pressure technique requires a third rescuer. The third rescuer can have no responsibility for rescue breathing or chest compressions. Only health-care professionals should use this technique and only when an extra rescuer is present. This means that during 2-rescuer CPR, 3 rescuers would actually be required: 1 rescuer to perform rescue breathing, 1 to perform chest compressions, and 1 to apply cricoid pressure.

To apply cricoid pressure (Figure 16),

- Locate the thyroid cartilage (Adam's apple) with your index finger.

- Slide your index finger toward the windpipe and feel for the "elevated area" below (cricoid cartilage).

- Using the tips of your thumb and index finger, apply firm backward pressure to this elevated area.

- Apply moderate rather than excessive pressure on the cricoid. Use of moderate pressure is particularly important if the victim is small.

FIGURE 16. Cricoid pressure (Sellick's maneuver).

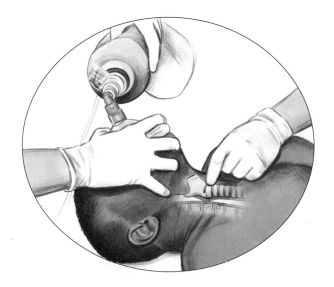

Foreign-Body Airway Obstruction

Foreign-body airway obstruction (FBAO), or choking, is an alarming and dramatic emergency. The desperate efforts of the choking person to clear his or her airway heighten the emotional drama and increase the pressure on the rescuer to take the correct action.

Victims with *severe or complete* FBAO will initially be responsive but will be unable to cough forcefully or speak. They may make high-pitched noises when they try to inhale. You must be prepared to relieve the obstruction with abdominal thrusts (the Heimlich maneuver).

To confirm a complete airway obstruction, ask the victim "Are you choking?" If the victim cannot speak or can make only weak, high-pitched sounds, perform abdominal thrusts until the object is expelled or the victim becomes unresponsive.

First Aid for Severe or Complete FBAO

Use abdominal thrusts (the Heimlich maneuver) to relieve severe or complete airway obstruction caused by a foreign body. Victims with severe or complete FBAO will be unable to cough forcefully or to speak. The victim may clutch the throat with one or both hands. Clutching the throat with one or both hands is called *the universal sign of choking* (Figure 17).

Abdominal thrusts (the Heimlich maneuver) quickly force air from the victim's lungs. This expels the blocking object like a cork from a bottle. Repeat abdominal thrusts until the object is expelled or the victim becomes unresponsive.

Sequence for Relief of FBAO in the *Responsive* Victim

If the choking victim is *responsive* and *standing*, use the following sequence to perform abdominal thrusts (the Heimlich maneuver) (Figure 17):

1. Stand behind the victim.

2. Make a fist with one hand.

3. Place your fist on the victim's abdomen, slightly above the navel and well below the breastbone.

4. Grasp your fist with your other hand.

5. Deliver quick upward thrusts into the victim's abdomen.

6. Deliver thrusts until the object is expelled or the victim becomes unresponsive.

If severe or complete FBAO is not relieved, the victim will stop breathing. If that happens the brain and heart

FIGURE 17. Abdominal thrusts (the Heimlich maneuver) for the responsive victim with severe or complete FBAO. If you see someone make the universal sign of choking (hands clutching the throat), perform abdominal thrusts. Stand behind the victim. Place the fist of one hand on the victim's abdomen, slightly above the navel but below the breastbone. Grasp your fist with your other hand. Use both hands to deliver quick upward thrusts. Deliver thrusts until the object is expelled or the victim becomes unresponsive.

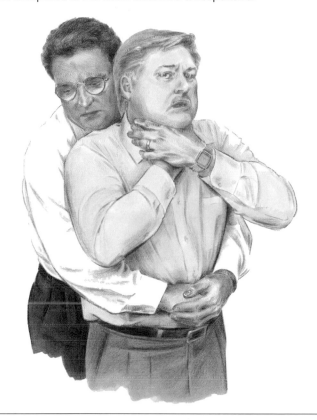

will not have enough oxygen. The victim will become unresponsive. When the victim becomes unresponsive and you are alone, *phone 911 (or other emergency response number) and get the AED.* Then begin the sequence for relief of FBAO in the unresponsive victim.

Sequence for Relief of FBAO in the *Unresponsive* Victim

Some victims of FBAO will be responsive when you find them and then become unresponsive. In this circumstance you will know that the cause of the victim's unresponsiveness is FBAO. Other victims of FBAO will be unresponsive when you find them. In this circumstance you will probably not know the victim has FBAO until repeated attempts at rescue breathing are unsuccessful.

Victims Who Become Unresponsive

If you see the victim collapse and you *know* FBAO is the cause, use the following sequence of actions:

- Phone 911 or the emergency response number. If a second rescuer is present, send that rescuer to phone 911 while you remain with the victim. Be sure the victim is lying on his or her back.

- Perform a tongue-jaw lift. Open the victim's mouth by grasping both the tongue and lower jaw between the thumb and fingers and lifting the mandible.

- Then sweep the victim's mouth with the index finger to remove the object (Figure 18).

- Open the airway and look, listen, and feel for adequate breathing. If the victim is not breathing adequately, give 1 or 2 rescue breaths. If the victim's chest does not rise with the breaths, reposition the head and give 1 or 2 more rescue breaths.

- If the victim's chest does not rise after you reposition the airway, kneel astride the victim's thighs (Figure 19) and perform abdominal thrusts. Give up to 5 thrusts and then repeat the sequence of tongue-jaw lift, finger sweep, attempt (and reattempt) to ventilate, and abdominal thrusts.

To deliver abdominal thrusts to the unresponsive victim:

- Kneel astride the victim's thighs. Place the heel of one hand against the victim's abdomen, in the midline slightly above the navel and well below the tip of the sternum (xiphoid).

- Place your second hand directly on top of the first. Press both hands into the abdomen with quick upward thrusts. Give 5 abdominal thrusts.

FIGURE 18. Tongue-jaw lift and finger sweep to relieve FBAO in an adult with severe or complete obstruction.

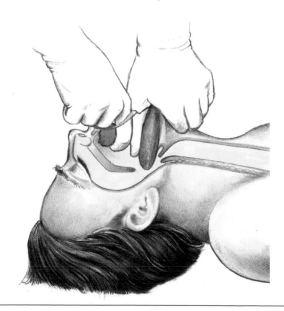

FIGURE 19. Abdominal thrusts for an unresponsive adult with severe or complete FBAO.

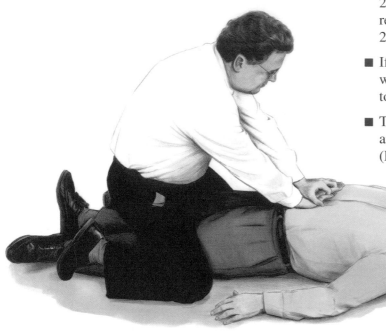

If you are in the correct position, you will be positioned over the middle of the abdomen. In this position you are unlikely to direct the thrusts to the right or left. Use the weight of your body to perform the maneuver.

Repeat the sequence of tongue-jaw lift, finger sweep, rescue breathing (attempt and reattempt), and abdominal thrusts until the obstruction is removed and the chest rises with rescue breaths, until the victim breathes adequately, or until advanced procedures are available to clear the airway.

Once you remove the obstruction, check breathing. If the victim is not breathing adequately, provide 2 slow rescue breaths. If the airway is clear (the obstruction has been completely removed), the chest will rise with each breath. Then check for signs of circulation (pulse, adequate breathing, coughing, or movement). If there are no signs of circulation, begin chest compressions and use the AED.

If the object is expelled during abdominal thrusts and you find the object in the pharynx when you perform the tongue-jaw lift, remove the object.

Victims Who Are Found Unresponsive

If you find an unresponsive person and do not know the cause of unresponsiveness, take these actions:

■ Phone 911 (or other emergency response number). If a second rescuer is present, send that rescuer to phone 911 while you stay with the victim.

■ Open the airway and check for breathing.

■ If the victim is not breathing adequately, give 1 or 2 rescue breaths. If the victim's chest does not rise, reposition the head (reopen the airway) and give 1 or 2 rescue breaths again.

■ If the chest does not rise after you reposition the airway, kneel astride the victim (Figure 19) and give up to 5 abdominal thrusts (the Heimlich maneuver).

■ Then open the victim's airway using a tongue-jaw lift and perform a finger sweep to remove the object (Figure 18).

■ Open the airway and give rescue breaths (reattempt if necessary). If the chest does not rise, give 5 abdominal thrusts.

Repeat the sequence of attempts (and reattempts) at rescue breathing, abdominal thrusts, and tongue-jaw lift and finger sweep until the obstruction is cleared, rescue breathing is effective, or advanced procedures are available to establish a clear airway.

If the obstruction is removed and the airway is cleared, check breathing. If the victim is not breathing, provide 2 rescue breaths. Then check for signs of circulation (pulse, adequate breathing, coughing, or movement). If there are no signs of circulation, begin chest compressions and use the AED. If the airway obstruction is cleared during abdominal thrusts, the victim may resume spontaneous breathing. If the victim does not resume spontaneous

FYI: FBAO in Pregnant and Obese Victims

If the choking victim is in the later stages of pregnancy or is obese, use chest thrusts instead of abdominal thrusts (Figure 20). Stand behind the victim and wrap your arms around the chest. Position your hands (one in a fist, the other grasping it) on the chest in the center of the sternum (breastbone) between the nipples. Deliver quick upward thrusts until the object is expelled or the victim becomes unresponsive.

If the victim becomes unresponsive, follow the sequence for the victim who becomes unresponsive. Be sure to use chest thrusts instead of abdominal thrusts. In the unresponsive pregnant or obese victim, chest thrusts are delivered in the same location and manner as chest compressions.

FIGURE 20. Chest thrusts to relieve severe or complete FBAO in the pregnant victim.

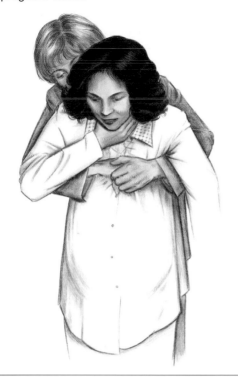

breathing, be prepared to provide as much rescue support as the victim requires.

Keeping Your Skills Sharp: CPR Practice

Review the steps and skills of 1-rescuer and 2-rescuer CPR regularly (several times every year). You can review the steps of CPR with practice videos and CPR prompt devices that give recorded instructions. Take an instructor-led refresher course at least every 2 years to maintain your CPR skills.

Never practice CPR skills on another person. Chest compressions can be lifesaving for a victim of cardiac arrest, but they can injure a responsive, healthy person.

Summary

The ABCs are an important set of skills that everyone should learn. As a healthcare provider you are likely to use these skills while caring for patients. In your lifetime you will probably encounter at least one emergency outside the healthcare facility. Your ability to perform CPR will help save a life or prevent an urgent problem from becoming a life-threatening emergency.

A: **A**irway problems are common. Everyone should know how to

- Open the airway of an unresponsive victim (head tilt–chin lift or jaw thrust)

- Use abdominal thrusts to relieve choking in a responsive victim

B: **B**reathing problems can occur during these emergencies:

- Respiratory and cardiac arrest

- FBAO (choking)

- Strokes and seizures

- Head trauma

- Drowning and near-drowning

- Medication overdose and drug intoxication

To manage breathing problems, you must know how to open the airway and give rescue breaths. As a healthcare provider you must be able to give rescue breaths with and without barrier and bag-mask devices. You must also know how to provide rescue breaths with a face mask or bag mask with and without oxygen.

C: **C**irculation problems may be present. Support circulation with *chest compressions* if the victim has no signs of circulation. Be prepared to use the AED (see Chapter 3) if there are no signs of circulation. The victim of cardiac arrest is unresponsive, is not breathing adequately, and has no signs of circulation in response to rescue breaths.

The most common cause of sudden adult cardiac arrest is VF. Chest compressions are simple and easy to learn and will "buy time" for the victim of cardiac arrest until defibrillation is performed.

Learning Checklist

Review the key information you learned in this chapter.

🗸 When you find an unresponsive victim:

- Phone 911 (or other emergency response number) and get the AED

- Open the airway and check breathing

- Give 2 slow rescue breaths if the victim is not breathing normally

- Check for signs of circulation

- If no signs of circulation are present, start chest compressions and be prepared to use the AED

🗸 **Airway and Breathing:** Open the victim's airway using the head tilt–chin lift (use the jaw thrust if a head or neck injury is present). Then look, listen, and feel for breathing.

■ Place your ear next to the victim's mouth and nose and look at the chest:

— **Look** for the chest to rise.

— **Listen** for breathing

— **Feel** for air movement on your cheek

■ If the victim is not breathing adequately, **give 2 slow rescue breaths (2 seconds each)**

■ Be sure the chest rises with each breath. If the chest does not rise, reopen the airway and give rescue breaths again.

✔ You can use a face shield, face mask, or bag-mask device to give rescue breaths. When you use a face mask or bag-mask device, you must achieve an air-tight seal. Use of a bag-mask device is easier and more effective with 2 rescuers.

✔ Cricoid pressure (Sellick's maneuver) prevents air from entering the stomach and aspiration of stomach contents into the lungs.

✔ Check for signs of circulation (pulse, adequate breathing, coughing, or movement in response to the 2 rescue breaths). If there are no signs of circulation, begin chest compressions. Deliver compressions at a rate of 100 compressions per minute.

✔ During 1- and 2-rescuer CPR the compression-ventilation ratio (number of compressions and number of breaths in a cycle) is 15:2. Continue cycles of 15 compressions and 2 breaths until a tracheal tube is inserted. Once a tube is inserted, give about 100 compressions per minute and 12 to 15 breaths per minute.

✔ Provide CPR for 1 minute and then recheck for signs of circulation. If there are no signs of circulation, continue CPR and check for signs of circulation every few minutes.

✔ Place a victim who is unresponsive but breathing with signs of circulation in the recovery position.

✔ Perform the Heimlich maneuver (abdominal thrusts) for responsive victims with signs of severe or complete FBAO. Place the fist just above the navel and well below the breastbone.

✔ If a victim with FBAO becomes unresponsive, phone 911 (or other emergency response number). Then perform the following sequence: tongue-jaw lift, finger sweep, rescue breathing, and abdominal thrusts (use chest thrusts for pregnant or obese victims). Repeat this sequence until the object is removed or personnel capable of providing advanced care arrive.

Review Questions

1. A patient suddenly collapses while undergoing an x-ray procedure. You gently shake him and shout "Are you OK?" but he does not respond. You are alone so you shout for help. What do you do if no one responds to your shout? (Choose the answer with the correct steps listed in the correct order.)

   a. call the emergency response number (and get the AED), return to the victim, check for signs of circulation (including a pulse), open the airway, check for breathing, and give 2 breaths if the victim is not breathing

   b. open the airway, give 2 breaths if the victim is not breathing, check for signs of circulation, and call the emergency response number and get the AED

   c. call the emergency response number and get the AED, return to the victim, open the airway, check for breathing, give 2 breaths (if victim is not breathing), and check for signs of circulation

   d. give 2 breaths (if victim is not breathing), check for signs of circulation, call 911 (and get the AED if available), return to the victim and begin chest compressions

2. You hear a patient cry out in the next room. You enter the room and find him collapsed on the floor. What is your first action?

   a. check for breathing

   b. check for signs of circulation

   c. check for responsiveness

   d. open the airway

3. You are alone when you find your 68-year-old patient lying unresponsive on the floor. You phone the emergency response number and grab the face mask in the room. You perform a head tilt–chin lift and look, listen, and feel for breathing. She is not breathing. What do you do next?

   a. give 2 rapid breaths using the face mask

   b. give 2 slow breaths using the face mask

   c. begin chest compressions, leaving the face mask on the victim's face

   d. place your patient in the recovery position

4. A patient at a clinic complains of chest discomfort, turns pale, and collapses. You determine that she is unresponsive, and you ask a colleague to phone the emergency response number and get the AED. You perform a head tilt–chin lift and look, listen, and feel for breathing. The patient is not breathing, so you give 2 rescue breaths. The chest rises with each breath. You then check for signs of circulation. Which of the following are the signs of circulation you should look for?

   a. a pulse or a response to the rescue breaths (adequate breathing, coughing, or movement)

   b. slow, gasping, irregular breaths

   c. blue, cool skin

   d. universal choking sign

5. The patient described in Question 4 has no signs of circulation. You begin chest compressions and then provide cycles of compressions and breaths. What is the correct ratio of compressions (pumping) to rescue breaths (blowing) that you should perform until the victim is intubated?

   a. 15 compressions to 2 breaths

   b. 10 compressions to 2 breaths

   c. 5 compressions to 2 breaths

   d. 5 compressions to 1 breath

6. A coworker collapses on the floor in the hospital cafeteria. You determine that she is unresponsive and ask a coworker to phone the emergency response number and get the AED. You perform a head tilt–chin lift and then look, listen, and feel for breathing. You detect no breathing, so you deliver 2 rescue breaths. What do you look for to determine whether your rescue breaths are effective?

   a. a change in the color of the victim's skin

   b. blueness of the lips

   c. rising of the chest during rescue breathing

   d. a snoring noise during exhalation

7. While you are eating in a cafeteria you see an elderly man suddenly clutch his throat. He cannot cough, and he nods his head yes when you ask if he is choking. He cannot speak. You tell him you are going to help him. What should you do immediately?

   a. perform head tilt–chin lift

   b. give several back blows

   c. give abdominal thrusts

   d. phone 911 or other emergency response number

How did you do?

1, c; 2, c; 3, b; 4, a; 5, a; 6, c; 7, c.

You work in a hospital. You have been asked to bring the code cart and the AED to a patient's room. On arriving in the room you see a 52-year-old man lying on the floor. CPR is in progress. One nurse is providing bag-mask ventilation, and another is providing chest compressions. The nurses in the room ask you to operate the AED. They confirm that the victim is unresponsive, is not breathing, and has no pulse or other signs of circulation.

You place the AED beside the victim's left ear, turn it on, and attach the electrodes to the victim. You "clear" the victim, and then you prompt the AED to analyze the victim's heart rhythm. The AED advises a shock. You again clear the victim and then deliver a shock. After the shock the AED again analyzes the rhythm. This time the AED gives a *"no shock advised"* message. The nurse at the victim's head verifies that he has a pulse and is moving slightly. Within seconds the victim begins to breathe adequately. The code team arrives and assumes responsibility for care of the victim.

You later learn that the victim was taken to the electrophysiology suite. He underwent extensive testing, and the treating physician implanted a cardioverter-defibrillator to help control the victim's heart rhythm. You visit the victim that evening and meet his wife and 2 children. They thank you for your immediate and appropriate actions.

Automated External Defibrillators (AEDs)

Overview

The most common cause of sudden cardiac arrest is an abnormal heart rhythm called *ventricular fibrillation* (VF). When VF develops, the rhythm of the heart becomes chaotic and the heart is unable to pump blood. The treatment for VF is *defibrillation* with a medical device called a *defibrillator*. A defibrillator delivers a shock to the heart. The shock interrupts the chaotic rhythm and allows the normal rhythm to resume. The time from collapse to defibrillation is the most important determinant of survival from sudden cardiac arrest. The shorter the time between collapse and defibrillation, the greater the victim's chance of survival.

AEDs are computerized defibrillators. These defibrillators are reliable and easy to operate, and they can be used by anyone with a few hours of training. Lay rescuer AED programs are a public health initiative that place AEDs throughout the community for use by trained lay rescuers. The goals of lay rescuer AED programs are to shorten the time to defibrillation for victims of cardiac arrest and to increase the rate of survival from cardiac arrest. Lay rescuer AED programs are the greatest advance in the treatment of cardiac arrest caused by VF since the development of CPR. Flight attendants, security personnel, police officers, firefighters, lifeguards, family members and many other trained lay rescuers have used AEDs successfully. AEDs are now available in many airports, airplanes, casinos, office buildings, housing complexes, recreational facilities, shopping malls, golf courses, and other public locations. Rescuers trained to use

Learning Objectives

After reading this chapter and practicing the skills you will be able to

1. Discuss the importance of early defibrillation

2. Discuss lay rescuer AED programs

3. Explain the purpose of an AED

4. List the 4 common steps required to operate all AEDs

5. Describe how to attach the AED electrode pads in the correct positions on the victim's chest

6. Explain why no one should touch the victim while the AED is analyzing, charging, or shocking the victim

7. List the special conditions that might change your actions when you use an AED

8. Describe the actions to take when the AED indicates no shock is needed

9. List the 3 criteria that determine when you start chest compressions and use the AED

10. Describe the roles for 3 rescuers at the scene of a cardiac arrest with an AED

11. Demonstrate the actions to take, according to the AED treatment algorithm, in the following scenarios:

    ■ No shock advised, no pulse

    ■ Shock advised, single shock, return of pulse and breathing

    ■ Shock advised, 3 shocks in a row, CPR for 1 minute, return of pulse after the fourth shock

12. Describe how to maintain an AED

AEDs are also present in these locations. The healthcare profession has embraced PAD.

AEDs are used by BLS ambulance providers and in hospitals, dental clinics, and physicians' offices. Extraordinary survival rates of up to 49% have been achieved with the use of AEDs. This rate is twice as high as survival rates previously reported by the most effective emergency medical services (EMS) systems. Use of AEDs is now taught as a BLS skill in all American Heart Association (AHA) courses. This means that BLS skills now include the first 3 links in the AHA Chain of Survival: early access to the emergency response system, early CPR, and early defibrillation. The fourth link in the Chain of Survival, early advanced care, is provided by persons trained in advanced cardiovascular life support (ACLS).

Link Between Early Defibrillation and Survival From Cardiac Arrest

Early defibrillation is critical for victims of sudden cardiac arrest because

- The most frequent rhythm in sudden cardiac arrest is VF

- The most effective treatment for VF is defibrillation

- Defibrillation is most likely to be successful if it occurs within minutes of collapse (cardiac arrest)

- Defibrillation may be ineffective if it is delayed

Presence or absence of bystander CPR and the time to defibrillation determines the success of resuscitative attempts. If no CPR is performed, survival from VF cardiac arrest falls by 7% to 10% with each minute that defibrillation is delayed (Figure 1). A survival rate of 70% to 90% is expected for witnessed arrest if defibrillation occurs within 1 minute of collapse. The survival rate falls to about 50% if defibrillation occurs 5 minutes after collapse and to about 30% at 7 minutes after collapse. The survival rate is only about 10% if defibrillation occurs 9 to 11 minutes after collapse. After 12 minutes the rate of survival is 2% or less.

CPR affects the rate of survival from sudden cardiac arrest because CPR helps preserve functioning of the heart and brain. CPR also increases the time that the heart is likely to respond to a shock. For this reason you must start CPR immediately and continue performing it until the AED arrives.

The sooner defibrillation occurs, the greater the victim's chance of survival from cardiac arrest. The AHA recommends the following goals for delivery of shocks: (1) *outside the hospital,* first shock provided within 5

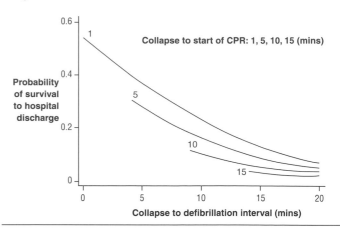

FIGURE 1. Relationship between time to defibrillation and success of resuscitation. The shorter the time to defibrillation, the greater the victim's chance of survival.

minutes after the call to the emergency response system; (2) *inside the hospital,* first shock provided within 3 minutes after collapse. Every community and healthcare facility should assess its ability to provide early defibrillation and establish whatever measures are needed to reach these goals.

Early defibrillation increases survival. Because of that fact, this link in the AHA Chain of Survival is now a standard part of BLS care. Widespread use of AEDs by the public and widespread availability of AEDs throughout the community significantly advance the concept proposed by the AHA more than 20 years ago: the community should become the "ultimate coronary care unit."

How AEDs Work

An AED is a computerized defibrillator (Figure 2) that

- Analyzes the heart rhythm

- Recognizes a "shockable" rhythm (a rhythm that is likely to respond to a shock)

- Advises the operator (through voice prompts and lighted buttons) whether the rhythm should be shocked

- Charges to the appropriate shock energy

You attach the AED to the victim with adhesive electrode pads. Once the electrodes are attached, the AED is able to analyze the victim's heart rhythm and determine if the rhythm is shockable. If a shock is needed, the AED charges to a preset energy level. When you press the SHOCK button, the AED delivers a shock to the victim through the electrodes.

FIGURE 2. AED attached to a victim.

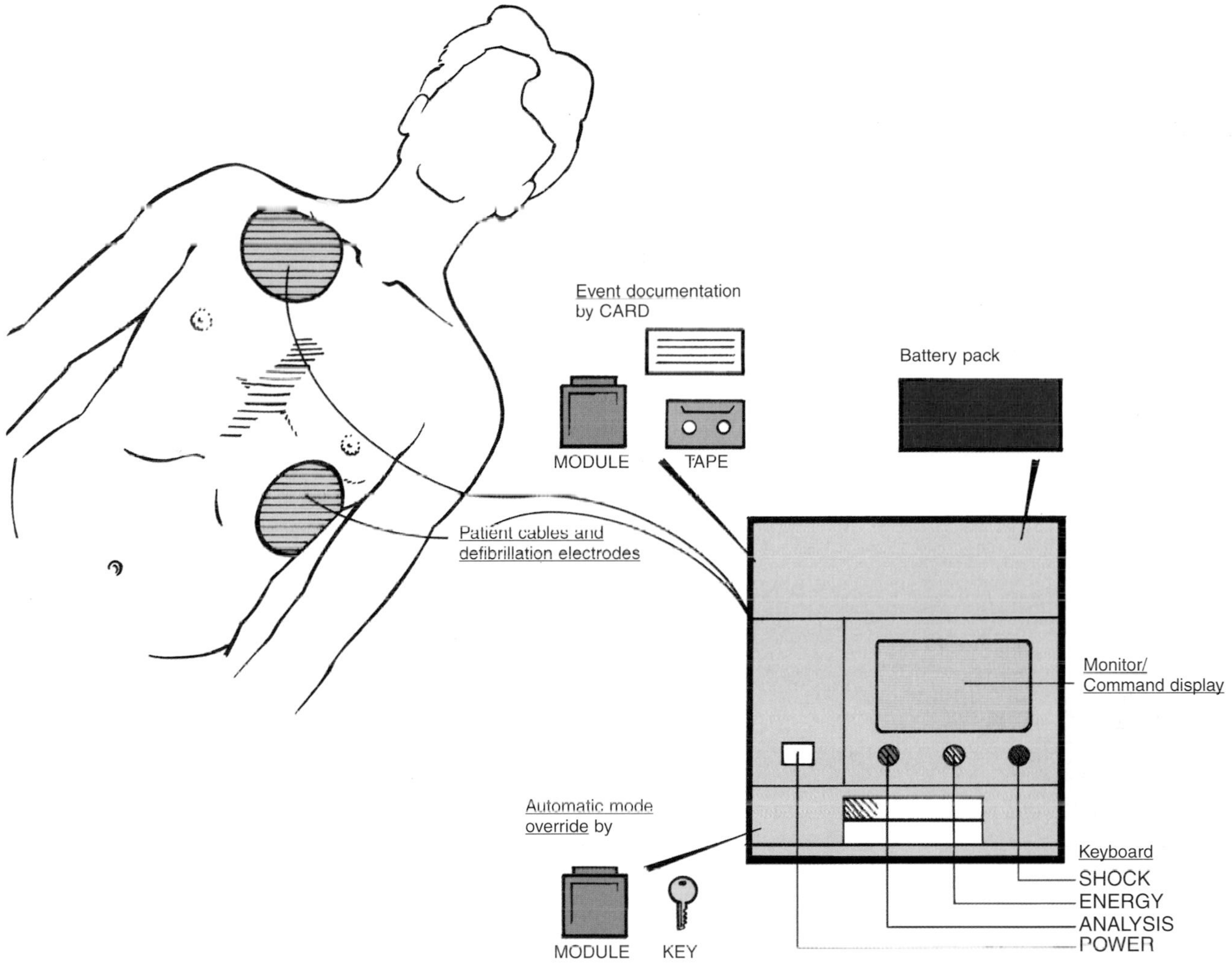

AEDs are relatively inexpensive and need little maintenance. They can be operated easily with little training. They are effective. For these reasons AEDs are now placed on airplanes and in public buildings, homes, and worksites. Many police officers carry AEDs in their cars, and are trained to perform CPR and use the AED. When many trained rescuers and many AEDs are available in a community, defibrillation is more likely to be provided within minutes of a cardiac arrest.

How an AED Analyzes the Heart Rhythm

AEDs contain computer chips that analyze the rate, size, and pattern of the victim's heart rhythm. AEDs are very accurate for use with adults.

AED electrodes have 2 functions:

■ To detect the electrical signal of the heart and send it to the computer for analysis

■ To deliver a shock if needed

AEDs analyze the victim's heart rhythm to determine if the rhythm is likely to respond to a shock, that is, if the rhythm is VF or ventricular tachycardia (VT). If a shockable rhythm (VF/VT) is identified, the AED will tell you (through a voice or lighted prompt) that a shock is advised. All AEDs must charge before they can deliver a shock. Some AEDs charge automatically. Others require that you press a CHARGE button. You then push another button to deliver the shock.

Operating an AED

Attach an AED only to a victim in cardiac arrest. Before you attach an AED, confirm that the 3 red flags of cardiac arrest are present:

1. No response

2. No adequate breathing

3. No signs of circulation (no adequate breathing, coughing, movement, or pulse)

Special Conditions That Affect the Use of AEDs

AEDs are accurate and safe to use in most situations. Nonetheless, 4 special conditions require you to change the way you use the AED: the victim is less than 8 years old, the victim is lying in water, the victim has an implanted medical device, or the victim has a medication patch. These conditions can result in harm to the victim or rescuer, and they can cause the AED to be ineffective. These conditions are discussed in the Critical Concepts box: "Special Conditions That Affect the Use of AEDs."

Placement of the AED

You must have enough room to perform CPR and operate the AED. Do not attempt CPR in a bed, for example, or with the victim slumped in a car or a chair. Place the victim on his back (supine) on a firm surface such as the floor. Place the AED so that the rescuer who will operate it can reach the AED controls easily, place the electrode pads in the proper locations, and direct CPR. If a second rescuer is providing CPR, place the AED on the side of the victim opposite the CPR rescuer, as close as possible to the victim. EMS rescuers should place the AED in the position that works best for them. Placement on the victim's left side is most convenient for electrode pad placement, so the left side is generally the best (but not the only) option.

The 4 Universal Steps of AED Operation

The AHA recommends that AEDs be stored next to a telephone. Storing the AED next to the phone allows the rescuer to call the emergency response number (or 911) and get the AED quickly.

Place the AED so that you can reach and operate the AED controls. If a second rescuer is providing CPR, put the AED on the side of the victim opposite the CPR rescuer.

AEDs are available in different models. The models differ slightly, but all AEDs operate in basically the same way. The 4 critical steps of AED operation are as follows:

Critical Concepts:
Special Conditions That Affect the Use of AEDs

1. **Children:** *Is the victim less than 8 years old?* AEDs may be used for children 1 to 8 years of age with no response, no normal breathing, and no signs of circulation after 1 minute of CPR. Use child pads if available. Do not use child pads on adult victims because they may not deliver enough energy for an adult. The AHA does not recommend for or against the use of AEDs in infants <1 years of age.

    Action:
    - Use the AED after 1 minute of CPR. Use child pads if available for victims less than 8 years of age.

2. **Water:** Is the victim's chest covered with water? A shock delivered to a victim in water could be conducted to the rescuers or bystanders. Water can also provide a path of energy from one AED pad to the other, bypassing the victim's heart.

    Actions:
    - If the victim's chest is covered with water, remove the victim from the water and quickly dry the chest before attaching AED electrodes.
    - If the victim is lying on snow or in a small puddle, you may use the AED if the chest is dry.

3. **Implanted pacemakers or defibrillators:** *Does the victim have a pacemaker or implanted cardioverter-defibrillator?* These devices are implanted in the upper part of the chest or abdomen (usually on the victim's left side). The devices create a hard lump beneath the skin. The lump is about half the size of a deck of cards. The victim will usually have a small scar. Placing an electrode pad over an implanted medical device will reduce the effectiveness of the shocks.

    Actions:
    - Do not place an AED electrode pad over an implanted device.
    - Place the electrode pad at least 1 inch to the side of the device.

4. **Transdermal medications:** *Does the victim have a medication patch on the chest where you would normally place the electrode pads?* Placing an AED electrode pad on top of a medication patch will prevent delivery of shocks or cause small burns to the skin.

    Action:
    - Remove the patch and wipe the area clean before attaching the AED.

Critical Concepts:
The 4 Universal Steps of AED Operation

1. *POWER ON* the AED.
2. *ATTACH* the electrode pads to the victim's chest.
3. Clear the victim and *ANALYZE* the heart rhythm.
4. Clear the victim and deliver a *SHOCK* (if indicated).

Step 1: POWER ON the AED

The first step in operating an AED is to *turn on the power*. Turning on the power starts the voice prompts, which will help you operate the AED. To turn on the AED, press the power switch, lift the monitor cover, or lift the screen to the "up" position.

Step 2: ATTACH the Adult Electrode Pads to the Victim's Chest

Quickly open the electrode package and remove the paper covering the adhesive backing. Attach the pads directly to the victim's chest. Some AEDs come with the pads, cables, and AED unit preconnected. All you do is attach the electrode pads to the victim's chest. Other devices may require you to connect the electrode cables and the AED unit or the cables and electrode pads (Figure 3). Four objects must be connected to attach the AED to the victim: AED unit→connecting cables→electrode pads→victim's chest.

FIGURE 3. The "AED-to-chest" circuit: AED unit→connecting cables→electrode pads→victim's chest.

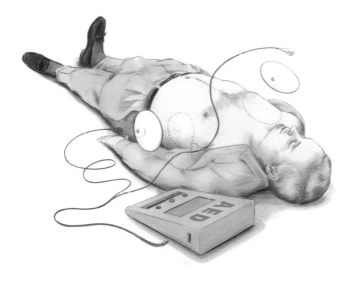

Place the first electrode pad in the *upper right* quadrant of the victim's chest. The proper location is next to the breastbone (sternum) between the nipple and the collarbone (clavicle). Remember: The victim's right side will be on *your left* side as you face the victim. Place the second pad outside the victim's left nipple (on *your right* side). Ensure that the top edge of the pad is several inches below the left armpit (Figure 4). The correct position of the electrode pads is often shown on the pads themselves or another part of the AED. The AED will work even if the pads are not placed exactly as pictured. Stop CPR just before you attach them (see Critical Concepts: Attaching AED Electrode Pads).

If the victim is extremely sweaty, dry the chest with a cloth or towel before you attach the electrode pads. Moisture can prevent the pads from sticking firmly to the chest.

Foundation Facts:
Making the Connections

AEDs require that 4 objects be connected in a line: the AED unit→connecting cables→electrode pads→and the victim's chest. To remember these 4 objects, begin at the AED unit and work your way to the victim:

1. The **AED** unit is joined to the
2. **Connecting cables,** which are joined to the
3. **Electrode pads,** which are joined to the
4. **Victim's chest**

Newer AEDs come with the AED unit, connecting cables, and electrode pads preconnected. All you do is open the electrode pad package, remove the paper covering the adhesive backing, and attach the pads to the victim's chest.

You will learn to operate an AED in this course. Ideally the AED you learn to operate will be the AED you will use in your workplace. AED manufacturers have not yet standardized these connections, so you must be familiar with the principles of AED operation to help you operate any AED. Before an emergency happens, learn exactly how much of the AED-to-chest circuit you must connect for the AED you will be using in your workplace. To figure out the connections that must be made, remember the 4 objects of the AED-to-chest circuit: **AED unit→ connecting cables→electrode pads→victim's chest** (Figure 3).

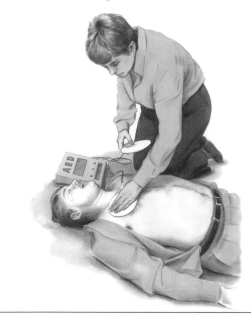

FIGURE 4. Attaching the AED.

If the victim has a hairy chest, the electrode pads may stick to the chest hair instead of the skin. If the electrode pads are not firmly attached to the skin, the AED will prompt you to *"check electrodes"* or *"check electrode pads."* To correct this problem, firmly press each pad. If the error message continues, briskly pull off the original pads. Pulling off the pads will remove the hair attached to them. Wipe the chest. If a lot of hair still remains where you will put the pads, shave the chest in the area of the pads, using the razor in the AED case. Then attach another set of electrode pads.

Step 3: Clear the Victim and ANALYZE the Heart Rhythm

With some AEDs you will need to press an ANALYZE button to start the analysis of the victim's heart rhythm. Other AEDs automatically begin analysis when the electrode pads are properly attached to the chest. "Clear" the victim (make sure no one is touching him) before analyzing the heart rhythm. Do not move the victim at all. Movement will interfere with the analysis. Rhythm analysis takes 5 to 15 seconds. If VF/VT is present, the AED will indicate that a shock is needed.

Step 4: Clear the Victim and Deliver a SHOCK (if Indicated)

Before you press the SHOCK button, make sure no one is touching the victim. Always loudly state a "clear the victim" message such as "I'm clear, you're clear, everybody's clear" or simply "Clear!" At the same time look to ensure that no one is in contact with the victim. *Do not let anyone touch the victim during analysis or delivery of shocks.* If anyone is touching the victim, do not push the ANALYZE or SHOCK button. A tone, voice message, or light will indicate when charging has started. Deliver a shock only after the victim is cleared. The shock will cause a sudden contraction of the victim's muscles.

After the first shock the AED should check the victim's rhythm again. Do not restart CPR at this time. Instead clear the victim and press the ANALYZE button. Some AEDs will automatically start another rhythm analysis cycle immediately after delivering a shock. In either case be sure that no one touches the victim immediately after the first shock. If VF/VT persists, the AED will indicate the need for another shock, and the *"charging"* and *"shock indicated"* sequence will repeat for the second (and possibly a third) shock.

After 3 shocks, check for signs of circulation (including a pulse). The goal is to deliver up to 3 shocks in rapid sequence if VF/VT is present and remains. If VF remains after 3 shocks, give CPR for 1 minute. Then attempt additional shocks. All AEDs will recommend that you check for signs of circulation after 3 shocks have been delivered even if VF/VT remains (see next section).

The universal steps for AED operation are reviewed in detail in Critical Concepts: The 4 Universal Steps of AED Operation.

Outcomes and Actions After Defibrillation

"Shock Indicated" Message: Recurrent VF/VT

Signs of Circulation Do Not Return After 3 Shocks

If signs of circulation do not return after 3 shocks and no ACLS providers have arrived, resume CPR for 1 minute. After 1 minute most AEDs will prompt you to check for signs of circulation. If the victim has no pulse or other signs of circulation and reanalysis indicates that VF/VT continues, deliver additional sets of up to 3 shocks. Follow the same procedure used for the first set of shocks: first shock, rhythm analysis, second shock (if indicated), rhythm analysis, third shock (if indicated), rhythm analysis, 1 minute of CPR (if no signs of circulation).

Shocks delivered in rapid sequence are called "stacked" shocks. Provide sets of up to 3 stacked shocks until the AED gives a *"no shock indicated"* message or until ACLS personnel arrive.

Do *not* check for signs of circulation between any two of the 3 stacked shocks in each set. For example, do not check for signs of circulation between shocks 1 and 2 or between shocks 2 and 3 of each set. *Do* check for signs of circulation after shock 3. Checking for signs of circulation between stacked shocks delays rapid identification of persistent VF/VT.

"No Shock Indicated"
No Signs of Circulation

When the AED gives a *"no shock indicated"* message, check for signs of circulation. If no signs of circulation (including a pulse) are present, resume CPR (chest compressions and rescue breathing). Three *"no shock indicated"* messages with no signs of return of circulation suggest that there is a low probability that the rhythm can be successfully defibrillated. If you receive 3 *"no shock indicated"* messages but find no signs of circulation, continue CPR and analyze the rhythm every 1 to 2 minutes. Remember to clear the victim before starting rhythm analysis.

Signs of Circulation Present

If signs of circulation (including a pulse) return, check breathing. If the victim is not breathing adequately, give 1 breath every 5 seconds (rescue breathing at a rate of 10 to 12 breaths per minute). If the victim is breathing adequately, place him in a recovery position. Leave the AED attached to the victim. If VF recurs, most AEDs will prompt the rescuer to check for signs of circulation. The device will then charge automatically and advise the rescuer to deliver an additional shock.

Using AEDs in a Moving Ambulance

Leave the AED attached to the victim during transport to the hospital. Do *not* push the ANALYZE button in a moving ambulance. Any movement of the victim, including movement caused by the ambulance, will interfere with rhythm analysis, and movement of the victim can simulate VF. Some AEDs analyze the victim's heart rhythm at regular and frequent intervals. Stop the vehicle if a victim requires rhythm analysis during transport or if the AED prompts the rescuer to check the victim or if the AED recommends a shock. Once the ambulance is completely stopped, clear the victim, analyze the rhythm, and deliver a shock if needed.

Use of an AED by 1 Rescuer

Sometimes only 1 rescuer can respond to a cardiac arrest. If you are the only rescuer at the scene of a cardiac arrest, do the following:

1. Verify unresponsiveness.
2. Phone the emergency response number and get the AED.
3. Return to the victim, open the airway, and check for breathing.
4. If the victim is not breathing adequately, give 2 rescue breaths.
5. Check for signs of circulation (including a pulse). If no signs of circulation are present, begin the steps of defibrillation (see the AED treatment algorithm).

Reasonable variations in this sequence are acceptable.

Integrating CPR and Use of the AED
When to Start CPR, When to Use the AED

There are 3 major signs (red flags) of cardiac arrest. These 3 signs are the cues for providing chest compressions and using the AED. Remember these 3 signs and be prepared to provide CPR (cycles of chest compressions and rescue breathing) and use the AED. The 3 red flags of cardiac arrest and the appropriate response to each are

- **No response:** Call 911 (or emergency response number) and get the AED.
- **No adequate breathing:** Give rescue breaths.
- **No signs of circulation:**
  — Start chest compressions
  — Use the AED

Once the AED is turned on, attached to the victim, and placed in analyze mode, it will identify 1 of 2 conditions. *"shockable rhythm present"* (shock advised or shock

---

Critical Concepts:
Unresponsive? Phone 911 and Get the AED!

Check unresponsiveness: Shout *"Are you OK?"*

If the victim does not respond:

Call 911 (or emergency response number) and get the AED. If another person is present, tell that person to call 911 and get the AED while you begin CPR.

The AED should be located next to the telephone.

indicated) or *shockable rhythm absent* (no shock advised or no shock indicated). If the AED advises a shock, clear the victim and press the SHOCK button. Once the AED indicates that no shock is advised, check for signs of circulation. If no signs of circulation are present, provide CPR (chest compressions and rescue breathing). If signs of circulation are present but breathing is absent or inadequate, provide rescue breathing. If adequate breathing *and* signs of circulation are present, place the victim in a recovery position.

Action Sequence: The AED Protocol

When you see a person who may be in cardiac arrest, act quickly but calmly. Follow the same sequences you learned for CPR and operation of the AED. To integrate CPR with use of an AED, you must learn

- The steps of CPR

- The steps of AED operation

- The full action sequence of the AED protocol

When you arrive at the scene of a suspected cardiac arrest, you must immediately activate the emergency response system and get the AED, provide CPR, and use the AED. In most situations additional rescuers will be present to help you.

In general, 3 actions must occur simultaneously at the scene of a cardiac arrest:

- Activate the emergency response system (and get the AED)

- Perform CPR

- Use the AED

When 2 or more rescuers are present, these actions are performed *simultaneously* rather than *sequentially*. For

example, one rescuer activates the emergency response system and gets the AED while another rescuer begins CPR. When the first rescuer returns with the AED, the AED is attached to the victim.

Practice scene leadership and team management during scenario and peer practice sessions. When more than 1 rescuer is present, there may be some confusion about the actions each rescuer should perform.

Sequence of Action for Use of an AED by 2 Rescuers

1. **Verify unresponsiveness:**
   If unresponsive:

   - Phone the emergency response number (or 911).

   - Get the AED (located next to the telephone).

     — The person who phones the emergency response number gets the AED.

     — The second rescuer stays with the victim and performs CPR until the AED arrives. In many circumstances the person who performs CPR also operates the AED, but rescuers can adjust these roles based on their skill and comfort level.

2. **Open airway:** Perform a head tilt–chin lift (use a jaw thrust if a head or neck injury is suspected).

Critical Concepts:
Red Flags of Cardiac Arrest

The 3 red flags of cardiac arrest in adults are

1. No response

2. No adequate breathing

3. No signs of circulation (no adequate breathing, no coughing, no movement, and no pulse)

If the victim has these 3 signs, begin chest compressions and provide cycles of compressions and rescue breathing and use the AED.

Critical Concepts:
The CPR-AED Protocol (ABCD)

Once you verify that a victim is unresponsive, phone 911 and get the AED. Then begin the CPR-AED protocol (ABCD).

A: Airway: Open the airway. Use the head tilt–chin lift or jaw thrust.

B: Breathing: Look, listen, and feel for breathing. Give 2 breaths if needed.

C: Circulation: Check for signs of circulation. Begin chest compressions if needed.

D: Defibrillation: The 4 universal steps of AED operation are

1. **POWER ON** the AED.

2. Attach the AED to the victim's chest.

3. Clear the victim and analyze the heart rhythm.

4. Clear the victim and deliver a shock (if indicated).

FIGURE 5. Two-rescuer CPR with use of an AED. The rescuer who gets the AED places it beside the victim's left ear.

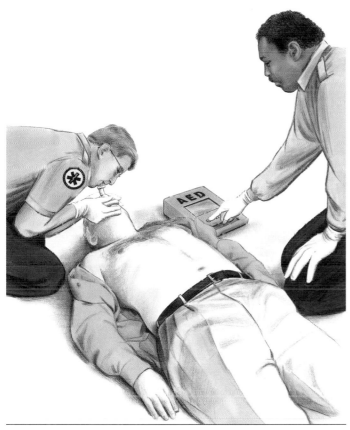

FIGURE 6. Two-rescuer CPR with use of AED. Operator turns on the AED.

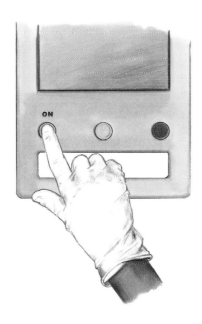

3. **Check breathing: If breathing is inadequate, provide rescue breathing.**

   ■ Check for breathing (*look, listen,* and *feel*).

   ■ If breathing is inadequate, give 2 slow breaths.

      — A face shield is most likely to be available outside the hospital.

      — A mouth-to-mask device (face mask) should be available in the AED carrying case.

      — A bag-mask device should be available in the healthcare facility.

4. **Check for signs of circulation:** If no signs of circulation are present:

   ■ Perform CPR (cycles of compressions and ventilations 15:2) and attach the AED.

      — If there is any doubt about the presence of signs of circulation, one rescuer performs CPR while the other rescuer prepares to use the AED.

      — Remove clothing covering the victim's chest to provide chest compressions and attach the AED electrode pads.

5. **Use the AED to provide defibrillation:** If no signs of circulation are present:

   ■ The caller delivers the AED to the rescuer performing CPR. Place the AED near the rescuer who will be using it (Figure 5). The AED is usually placed on the side of the victim opposite the rescuer who is performing CPR.

   ■ Actions for the AED operator:

   — **POWER ON** the AED and follow voice prompts. Some devices will turn on when the AED lid or carrying case is opened (Figure 6).

   — **ATTACH** the AED to the victim (Figure 7):

      ● Select the correct pads for victim's size and age (adult vs child).

      ● Peel the backing from the pads.

      ● Attach the adhesive pads to the victim's bare chest. Just before you attach the pads to the victim's chest, tell the rescuer to stop chest compressions.

      ● Attach the electrode cable to the AED (if not preconnected).

FIGURE 7. Attaching the AED to the victim.

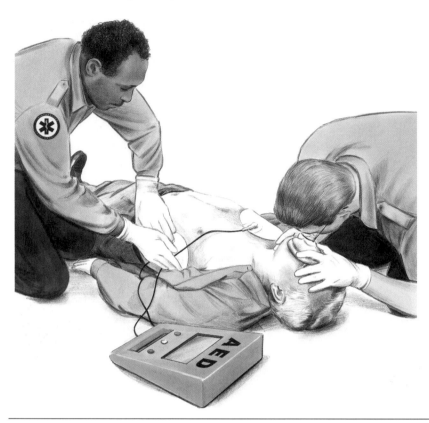

— **ANALYZE** the heart rhythm (Figure 8):

- Clear the victim before and during analysis.

- Check that no one is touching the victim (clear the victim).

- Press the ANALYZE button to start rhythm analysis (some AEDs automatically start analysis when the pads are properly attached to the victim).

— **Deliver a SHOCK (if indicated)** (Figure 9A and 9B).

- Clear the victim (loudly state "I'm clear, you're clear, oxygen's clear, everybody's clear").

- Check that no one is touching the victim.

- Press the SHOCK button (the victim's muscles may contract).

    ◆ Clear the victim and press the ANALYZE button (if necessary).

FIGURE 8. Analysis of the victim's heart rhythm. **A,** Operator clears the victim before rhythm analysis. **B,** Operator then presses the ANALYZE button if necessary.

A

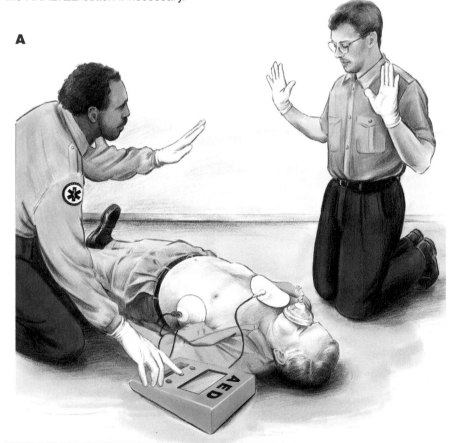

B

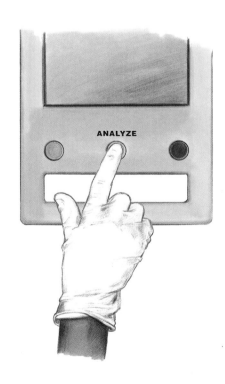

FIGURE 9. Delivery of shocks. **A,** Operator clears the victim before delivering a shock. **B,** Operator then presses the SHOCK button.

A

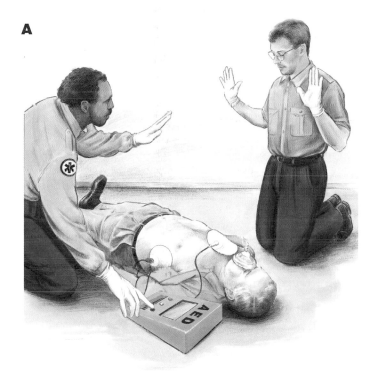

B

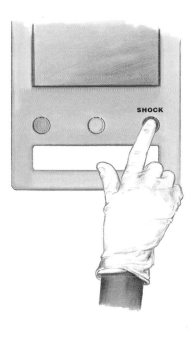

FIGURE 10. If the AED gives a *"no shock indicated"* message, check for signs of circulation (including a pulse).

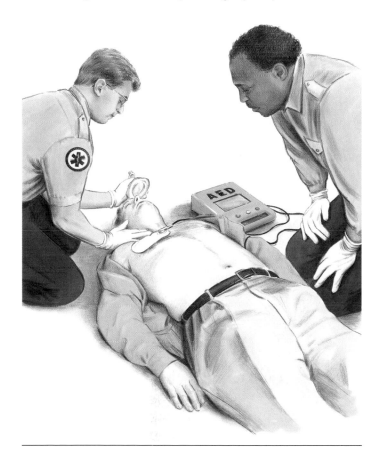

♦ Deliver up to 2 more shocks. (Press the SHOCK button up to 2 more times — 3 shocks total if the AED signals *"shock advised"* or *"shock indicated"* after each analysis. Clear the victim before each analysis and shock.)

— *"No shock indicated"* message (Figure 10):

● Check for signs of circulation (including a pulse). If signs of circulation are present, check breathing:

♦ If breathing is inadequate, provide rescue breathing.

♦ If breathing is adequate, place the victim in a recovery position and leave the AED attached.

● If no signs of circulation are present, resume CPR for 1 minute and then recheck for signs of circulation.

♦ If there are still no signs of circulation, analyze the rhythm and follow the *"shock indicated"* or *"no shock indicated"* steps as appropriate.

Critical Concepts:
"Shock" Messages and Related Actions

After the AED analyzes the heart rhythm, it will give you 1 of 2 possible messages: *"shock indicated"* or *"no shock indicated."* Depending on the AED, the message may say *"shock advised"* or *"no shock advised."*

- If the AED gives a *"shock indicated"* or *"shock advised"* message, clear the victim and then press the SHOCK button.

- If the AED indicates *"no shock indicated"* or *"no shock advised,"* check for signs of circulation (including a pulse). Be prepared to provide CPR.

- If no signs of circulation are found, resume CPR for 1 minute. Then recheck for signs of circulation.

- If no signs of circulation are found a second time, clear the victim and analyze the victim's rhythm again.

- After 3 *"no shock indicated"* messages, resume CPR and analyze the victim's rhythm every 1 to 2 minutes. Be sure to clear the victim before you analyze the rhythm.

Caring for the Victim After Successful Defibrillation

When signs of circulation and breathing return, place the patient in a recovery position. Leave the AED electrodes attached to the victim and the AED. Leave the AED turned on. Continue to monitor the victim. Many AEDs monitor the victim's heart rhythm at regular and frequent intervals. These AEDs will indicate if VF/VT recurs. Frequently check the victim for breathing and signs of circulation.

Lay rescuer AED programs should coordinate with the on-site ACLS team or local EMS system to ensure seamless transfer of care to appropriate BLS or ACLS healthcare providers after use of an AED.

Figure 11 is the AED treatment algorithm. This algorithm summarizes the steps for treatment of a victim of cardiac arrest and use of the AED before the arrival of ACLS personnel.

AED Maintenance and Troubleshooting

Newer AEDs require almost no maintenance. They are programmed to run self-tests, and they will indicate when maintenance is needed. You and your coworkers who are trained to use an AED must still ensure that your AED is ready for use at a moment's notice (see Critical Concepts box, AED Maintenance).

AED manufacturers provide specific recommendations for maintenance and AED readiness checks. Refer to the *manufacturer's instructions* and *guide to maintenance* in the AED carrying case, your PAD program manual, or the reference material at the medical center where you work. Your course instructor will give you information about AED maintenance. If you need more information, your instructor will refer you to an appropriate source. If instructions from the manufacturer are unavailable, use the sample checklists in Tables 1 and 2.

Critical Concepts:
AED Maintenance

- Become familiar with your AED and how it operates.

- Check the AED for visible problems such as signs of damage.

- Check the *"ready-for-use"* indicator on your AED (if so equipped) daily.

- Perform all user-based maintenance according to the manufacturer's recommendations.

- Make sure the AED carrying case contains the following supplies at all times:

  — 2 sets of extra electrode pads (3 sets total)

  — 2 pocket face masks

  — 1 extra battery (if appropriate for your AED; some AEDs have batteries that last for years)

  — 2 disposable razors (supplied by the manufacturer)

  — 5 sterile gauze pads (4 × 4 inches), individually wrapped

  — 1 absorbent cloth towel

Remember: AED malfunctions are rare. Most AED "problems" are caused by operator error or failure to perform recommended user-based maintenance.

FIGURE 11. AED treatment algorithm for out-of-hospital use of AEDs.

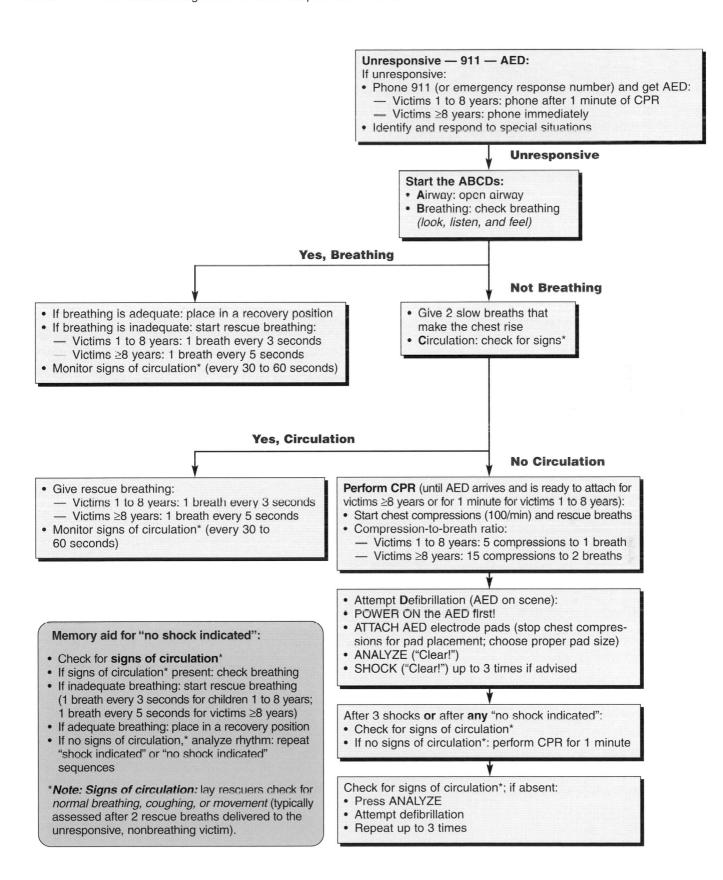

Unresponsive — 911 — AED:
If unresponsive:
- Phone 911 (or emergency response number) and get AED:
  — Victims 1 to 8 years: phone after 1 minute of CPR
  — Victims ≥8 years: phone immediately
- Identify and respond to special situations

Unresponsive

Start the ABCDs:
- **A**irway: open airway
- **B**reathing: check breathing *(look, listen, and feel)*

Yes, Breathing

Not Breathing

- If breathing is adequate: place in a recovery position
- If breathing is inadequate: start rescue breathing:
  — Victims 1 to 8 years: 1 breath every 3 seconds
  — Victims ≥8 years: 1 breath every 5 seconds
- Monitor signs of circulation* (every 30 to 60 seconds)

- Give 2 slow breaths that make the chest rise
- **C**irculation: check for signs*

Yes, Circulation

No Circulation

- Give rescue breathing:
  — Victims 1 to 8 years: 1 breath every 3 seconds
  — Victims ≥8 years: 1 breath every 5 seconds
- Monitor signs of circulation* (every 30 to 60 seconds)

Perform CPR (until AED arrives and is ready to attach for victims ≥8 years or for 1 minute for victims 1 to 8 years):
- Start chest compressions (100/min) and rescue breaths
- Compression-to-breath ratio:
  — Victims 1 to 8 years: 5 compressions to 1 breath
  — Victims ≥8 years: 15 compressions to 2 breaths

- Attempt **D**efibrillation (AED on scene):
- POWER ON the AED first!
- ATTACH AED electrode pads (stop chest compressions for pad placement; choose proper pad size)
- ANALYZE ("Clear!")
- SHOCK ("Clear!") up to 3 times if advised

Memory aid for "no shock indicated":

- Check for **signs of circulation***
- If signs of circulation* present: check breathing
- If inadequate breathing: start rescue breathing (1 breath every 3 seconds for children 1 to 8 years; 1 breath every 5 seconds for victims ≥8 years)
- If adequate breathing: place in a recovery position
- If no signs of circulation,* analyze rhythm: repeat "shock indicated" or "no shock indicated" sequences

***Note: Signs of circulation:** lay rescuers check for normal breathing, coughing, or movement* (typically assessed after 2 rescue breaths delivered to the unresponsive, nonbreathing victim).

After 3 shocks **or** after **any** "no shock indicated":
- Check for signs of circulation*
- If no signs of circulation*: perform CPR for 1 minute

Check for signs of circulation*; if absent:
- Press ANALYZE
- Attempt defibrillation
- Repeat up to 3 times

TABLE 1. Example of Checklist for AED Readiness. The checklist may be individualized for specific AED use.

Readiness-for-Use Checklist: Automated External Defibrillators for Healthcare Providers: Daily/Weekly Checklist

Organization Name/Identifier _____ **Mfr/Model No.** _____ **Serial/ID No.** _____

Date _____ **Covering Period** _____ **to** _____

At the beginning of each shift or at the scheduled time, inspect the device using the checklist below. Note any inconsistencies, deficiencies, and corrective actions taken. If the device is not ready for use or is out of service, write OOS on the "day of month" line and note deficiencies in the corrective action log.

Corrective Action Log

Day of Month/Signature/Unit No.

1. **Defibrillator unit**
   a. Clean, no spills, unobstructed
   b. Casing intact
2. **Defibrillation cables and connectors**
   a. Inspect for cracks, broken wires, or damage
   b. Connectors engage securely
3. **Supplies available**
   a. Two sets of unexpired hands-free defibrillator pads in sealed packages
   b. PPE — gloves, barrier device, or equivalent
   c. Razor and scissors
   d. Hand towel
   e. *Spare event documentation device
   f. *ECG paper
   g. *ECG monitoring electrodes
   h. *ALS module/key/equivalent
4. **Power supply**
   a. Verify fully charged battery(ies) in place
   b. *Spare charged battery available
   c. *Rotate batteries per manufacturer's specifications
   d. *AC power plugged into live outlet
5. **Indicators and screen display**
   a. *POWER ON display and self-test OK
   b. *ECG monitor display functional
   c. *No error or service required indicator/message
   d. Correct time displayed/set; synchronized with dispatch center
6. **ECG paper and event documentation device**
   a. *Event documentation device in place and functional
   b. *Adequate ECG paper
   c. *ECG recorder functional
7. **Charge/display cycle for defibrillation**
   a. Test per manufacturer's recommended test procedure
   b. *Identifies shockable rhythm
   c. *Charges to appropriate energy level
   d. *Acceptable discharge detected
8. **AED returned to patient ready status**

Day of Month: 1. 2. 3. 4. 5. 6. 7. 8. 9. 10. 11. 12. 13. 14. 15. 16. 17. 18. 19. 20. 21. 22. 23. 24. 25. 26. 27. 28. 29. 30. 31.

Example: 5. John Jones (signature)/Aid 2 checked Aid 2's device on the 5th day of this month and found it ready for use.

*Applicable only if the device has this capability/feature or if required by medical authorization.

TABLE 2. Example of a Readiness Checklist for Public Access Defibrillation With an AED. The checklist may be individualized.

Readiness-for-Use Checklist: Public Access Defibrillation With an AED
Date _____ **Covering Period** _____ **to** _____
*(This checklist can cover 1 month if **daily** check is used or 1 year if **monthly** check is used.)*

Organization Name/Identifier _____ **Mfr/Model No.** _____ **Serial/ID No.** _____

At the beginning of each shift or scheduled time, inspect the AED, using the checklist below. Note any inconsistencies, deficiencies, and corrective actions taken. If the device is not ready for use or out of service, write OOS on the "day of month" line and note deficiencies in the corrective action log.

Daily check:
1. Visually inspect the AED (if in "alarmed" holder):
   a. In proper location
   b. Clean, no spills
   c. No signs of tampering or inappropriate opening
   d. All readiness-for-use indicators, including battery, indicate "ready"

Monthly check (assuming no clinical uses):
2. Defibrillator cables and connectors
   a. Inspect for any outward signs of damage
   b. Engage/disengage connectors (pads to cables, cables to AED)
3. Supplies available
   a. 3 sets of unexpired hands-free defibrillator pads in sealed packages
   b. Personal protective equipment (gloves, barrier device)
   c. Razor and scissors
   d. Hand towel
   e. *Spare event documentation module ("Flash" card, PCMCIA card, magnetic storage)
4. Power supply
   a. Inspect battery-status display
   b. Verify AED signals "AED ready for use" or equivalent
   c. *AC power plugged into main if battery requires "trickle charge"
5. Indicators and screen display
   a. *POWER ON, self-test runs, display runs, verify OK
   b. *Monitor display functional
   c. *No "error" or "service required" indicator/message
   d. *Correct time displayed/set; synchronized with dispatch center/set
6. ECG event documentation module
   a. Follow manufacturer's recommendations
   b. *Event documentation module in place and functional
7. Charge/discharge cycle to simulated VF
   a. Perform charge/discharge test cycle per mfr's recommendations
   b. Input shockable rhythm (VF); use proper connection components
   c. *AED analysis identifies shockable rhythm
   d. *Charges to appropriate energy level
   e. *Acceptable discharge detected
8. AED returned to ready-for-use status

Day of Month/Signature/Unit No.

1. _____
2. _____
3. _____
4. _____
5. _____
6. _____
7. _____
8. _____
9. _____
10. _____
11. _____
12. _____
13. _____
14. _____
15. _____
16. _____
17. _____
18. _____
19. _____
20. _____
21. _____
22. _____
23. _____
24. _____
25. _____
26. _____
27. _____
28. _____
29. _____
30. _____
31. _____

Example: 5. John Jones (signature)/AED 2 checked on October 5 and found ready for use.

---

*Indicates features that vary greatly among AED brands and models. Applies only to devices with this capability or feature or if required by medical authority.

Corrective Action Log

_____
_____
_____
_____
_____
_____
_____
_____
_____
_____
_____

Month/Signature/Unit No.

January: _____
February: _____
March: _____
April: _____
May: _____
June: _____
July: _____
August: _____
September: _____
October: _____
November: _____
December: _____

Summary

The shorter the time between collapse from sudden cardiac arrest and defibrillation, the higher the victim's chance of survival. Early defibrillation is critical for both out-of-hospital and in-hospital sudden cardiac arrest. Lay rescuer AED programs provide the equipment and trained rescuers needed to defibrillate victims of out-of-hospital arrest within a few minutes of collapse. Such programs are the greatest advance in the treatment of cardiac arrest caused by VF since the development of CPR. Resuscitation programs in hospitals must also focus on shortening the time to defibrillation for victims of sudden cardiac arrest.

The AHA recommends the following goals for early defibrillation: outside the hospital, first shock provided within 5 minutes from the call to EMS to defibrillation; inside the hospital, first shock provided within 3 minutes from collapse to defibrillation. Every community and every emergency response system must assess its ability to provide early defibrillation and take whatever measures are necessary to make these goals a reality. Use of an AED is now taught as a BLS skill. After taking this course you will be able to provide the first 3 links in the Chain of Survival: early access, early CPR, and early defibrillation.

Learning Checklist

✔ The time between collapse and defibrillation is the greatest determinant of survival after sudden cardiac arrest. The shorter the time, the greater the victim's chance of survival.

✔ Lay rescuer AED programs make both AEDs and trained rescuers widely available throughout the community. Lay rescuer AED programs are the greatest advance in the treatment of victims of cardiac arrest since CPR.

✔ The purpose of an AED is to provide defibrillation as soon as possible to victims of VF. AEDs require little maintenance, are easy to use, and are accurate. AEDs can be used by lay rescuers and early responders.

✔ The 4 universal steps of AED operation are

1. **POWER ON** the AED

2. **ATTACH** the electrode pads to the victim's chest (stop chest compressions just before attachment)

3. Clear the victim and **ANALYZE** the heart rhythm

4. Clear the victim and deliver a **SHOCK** (if indicated)

Critical Concepts: The 4 Universal Steps of AED Operation

1. **POWER ON the AED.** This activates voice prompts that will help you operate the AED.
   - Open the carrying case or top of the AED.
   - Turn on the power. Some AEDs will start automatically when you open the lid or case.

2. **ATTACH electrode pads** to the victim's bare chest. Stop CPR just before you attach the pads.
   - Choose correct pad (adult vs child) for size/age of victim. Use child pads for children less than 8 years of age if available. Do not use child pads for an adult victim.
   - Peel the backing away from the electrode pads. Stop CPR.
   - Attach the adhesive electrode pads to the victim's bare chest.
   - Attach the AED connecting cables to the AED box (some are preconnected).

3. Clear the victim and **ANALYZE the heart rhythm.**
   - Clear the victim and press the ANALYZE button. Pressing the ANALYZE button will start rhythm analysis. Some AEDs will automatically begin analysis once the electrode pads are properly attached.
   - Always clear the victim before analysis. Be sure no one is touching the victim, not even the person in charge of rescue breathing.

4. Clear the victim and **deliver a SHOCK** (if indicated).
   - Clear the victim. Again make sure no one is touching the victim. Touching the victim during delivery of shocks may cause an ineffective shock to the victim, a shock to the person touching the victim, or burns on the victim or person touching him.
   - Press the SHOCK button to deliver a shock. Press the SHOCK button only when the AED indicates a shock is needed AND *only* when no one is touching the victim.

✔ The proper locations of the electrode pads are usually shown on the AED unit, the electrode pads, or the electrode packaging. Attach the pads directly to the victim's skin.

- Place 1 electrode pad in the upper right quadrant of the victim's chest (this will be on your left side as you face the victim). Make sure the pad is to the right of the victim's breastbone, between the nipple and the collarbone.

- Place the other electrode pad outside the left nipple. Make sure the top edge of the pad is several inches below the victim's left armpit.

✔ The AED operator must ensure that no one is touching the victim during the analyze, charging, and shock modes. Touching the victim during the analyze mode interferes with the interpretation of the victim's rhythm. The shock can be transferred to anyone touching the victim during the charging and shock modes.

✔ Four special conditions will require you to change how you use an AED:

1. The victim is less than 8 years old. Use an AED after 1 minute of CPR. Use child pads if available for children, but do not use child pads on adults.

2. The victim is lying in water. (Move the victim to a dry area and dry the chest.)

3. The victim has an implanted pacemaker or defibrillator. (Place the electrode pad away from the device.)

4. The victim has a transdermal medication patch. (Remove the patch and clean that area of the chest.)

✔ If the AED provides a *"no shock indicated"* message, perform the following actions:

1. Check for signs of circulation.

2. If signs of circulation are present, check breathing. If breathing is inadequate, provide rescue breathing.

Critical Concepts: Attaching AED Electrode Pads

Practice choosing the correct size (adult or child) AED electrode pads and opening the package while your partner performs CPR. When you are ready to attach the electrode pads to the victim, remove the sheet covering the adhesive backing of the first pad. Then ask your partner to stop CPR. Quickly press the pads onto the skin of the victim's chest. Then clear the victim and allow the AED to analyze the heart rhythm.

With some AEDs you will have to press the ANALYZE button. Other AEDs will automatically analyze the victim's rhythm as soon as the electrode pads are properly attached to the victim. You will receive an error message if the electrode pads are not firmly attached to the chest or if the cables are not properly connected. The message will be a voice warning or an alarm. The voice warning will state *"check pads," "check electrodes,"* or words to that effect. This warning means that there is a poor connection somewhere between the victim's chest and the AED.

Troubleshoot by performing the following checks:

1. If the victim has a hairy chest, the electrode pads may stick to the hair instead of the skin. This will lead to a *"check electrodes"* or *"check electrode pads"* message on the AED.

Try the following to solve this problem:

- Press firmly on each pad.

- If pressing the pads does not work, briskly pull the pads off the chest. This will remove chest hair. Wipe the chest. If a lot of hair remains where you pull off the pads, shave the area with the razor in the AED carrying case. Then attach a new set of pads. Professional responders use plastic disposable razors to shave the chest so that the electrode pads stick directly to the skin.

2. If the victim is wet or sweaty, remove the pads, wipe the chest dry with a cloth, and attach a new set.

3. Be sure the electrode pads stick firmly and evenly to the skin of the chest.

4. Check the cables to be sure they are properly connected to the electrode pads.

5. Check the cables to be sure they are properly connected to the AED unit.

Once you correct the problem, most AEDs will automatically begin to analyze the heart rhythm.

If breathing is adequate, place the victim in a recovery position. Leave the AED attached to the victim.

3. If there are no signs of circulation are present, resume CPR for 1 minute. Then recheck for signs of circulation.

4. If there are no signs of circulation after 1 minute of CPR, analyze the heart rhythm again.

5. Then follow the *"shock indicated"* or *"no shock indicated"* steps.

✔ The 3 criteria for determining when to start chest compressions and use the AED are the 3 red flags of cardiac arrest:

1. No response

2. No adequate breathing

3. No signs of circulation (no adequate breathing, no coughing, no movement, and no pulse)

✔ The role of cardiac arrest rescuers includes phoning the emergency response number (or 911), performing CPR, and attaching and using the AED.

Review Questions

1. You find an unresponsive adult. You send a colleague to phone the emergency response number and get the AED. You open the victim's airway and find that the victim is not breathing. You use a barrier device and deliver 2 breaths. The victim's chest rises with each breath. You check for signs of circulation. There are no signs of breathing, coughing, or movement, and you do not feel a carotid pulse. Your colleague has returned with the AED. He places it next to the victim's left ear and opens the case. Which of the following answers lists the 4 universal steps of AED operation in proper order?

    a. phone 911, begin CPR, use the AED, and provide advanced life support

    b. move the victim to a safe place, attach the electrode pads to the victim's chest, attach the cables to the electrode pads, and attach the cables to the AED

    c. check for signs of circulation, power on the AED, deliver a shock, and analyze the victim's rhythm

    d. power on the AED, attach the electrode pads to the victim's chest and the AED, clear the victim and analyze the heart rhythm, and clear the victim and deliver a shock if needed

2. You are assessing an unresponsive 52-year-old woman. You send a colleague to phone the emergency response number and get the AED. You open the victim's airway, check for breathing, and deliver 2 rescue breaths. Each breath makes her chest rise. You then check for signs of circulation and feel a strong, regular pulse. Nonetheless her face has turned blue, and she isn't breathing. What do you do next?

    a. attach the AED and start the shock cycle

    b. attach the AED, clear the victim, and analyze the heart rhythm

    c. provide rescue breathing

    d. attach the AED and monitor the heart rhythm

3. You see a middle-aged man clutch his chest and collapse. What are the 3 criteria for beginning CPR and using an AED for this person?

    a. no response, body movement, no breathing

    b. no response, coughing, no adequate breathing

    c. no response, body movement, weak breathing

    d. no response, no adequate breathing, no signs of circulation

4. You are alone and you see an adult suddenly collapse. Which is the correct sequence of actions for you to take?

    a. phone 911 or the emergency response number, verify unresponsiveness, perform the ABCDs

    b. phone 911 or the emergency response number, perform the ABCDs, verify unresponsiveness

    c. verify unresponsiveness, phone 911 or the emergency response number, perform the ABCDs

    d. verify unresponsiveness, perform the ABCDs for 1 minute, phone 911 or the emergency response number

5. You attach an AED to the chest of a 63-year-old man who is unresponsive, not breathing, and has no signs of circulation. After 3 shocks the AED gives you a *"no shock indicated"* message. You check the victim but he still has no signs of circulation. What do you do next?

    a. deliver a second set of 3 shocks

    b. press the ANALYZE button repeatedly until a shock is advised

    c. perform CPR (compressions and ventilations) for 1 minute, check for signs of circulation, and if no signs are present, press the ANALYZE button

    d. perform CPR until EMS or advanced care personnel arrive

6. You are treating a victim of cardiac arrest. You have turned on the AED, attached the electrode pads to the victim and the connecting cables to the AED, cleared the victim, and pressed the ANALYZE button. The AED analyzes the victim's heart rhythm, gives a *"shock indicated"* message, and charges to the appropriate level of energy. What do you do next?

    a. press the SHOCK button

    b. shout "clear!" and make sure no one is touching the victim

    c. press the ANALYZE button

    d. check for signs of circulation

How did you do?

1, d; **2,** c; **3,** d; **4,** c; **5,** c; **6,** b.

You are supervising a group of toddlers in a daycare center. You see a boy sitting among several toys in the play area. He appears to be breathing rapidly. You call his name. He looks at you, but he does not reply. You run to him, and you see that he is struggling to breathe. You hear a weak, high-pitched sound when he tries to inhale. You quickly give abdominal thrusts. On the third thrust a small toy is expelled from his mouth, and he begins to cry.

Is foreign-body airway obstruction (choking) a potential cause of cardiopulmonary arrest in a child? Could choking have been prevented in this scenario? How?

Prevention of Injuries and Arrest in Children and Infants

Overview

The first 3 chapters of this manual describe basic life support (BLS) and cardiopulmonary resuscitation (CPR) for adults. Chapters 4 and 5 describe BLS and CPR for infants (up to 1 year old) and children (1 to 8 years old). Throughout these chapters the terms *child*, *pediatric*, and *children* may be used to refer to this entire age group (from birth to 8 years old). Most of the injury prevention information is applicable to older children and adolescents.

Pediatric CPR and BLS must become part of the community-wide Chain of Survival. Making pediatric CPR and BLS part of the community-wide Chain of Survival will improve the chance of survival of all children after emergencies. The pediatric Chain of Survival includes prevention of cardiopulmonary arrest and injuries, early CPR, early access to the emergency response system, early advanced care, and postresuscitation and rehabilitative care.

AHA Chain of Survival for Infants and Children

In the United States the leading cause of death in infants during the first 6 months of life is SIDS. In older infants, children, and young adults, injuries are the leading cause of cardiac arrest and death. The most common causes of fatal injury in children and adolescents are motor vehicle crashes, drowning, burns, smoke inhalation, and firearms. Poisoning and choking are also common causes of death or disability in children. All of these causes can lead to breathing emergencies and cardiac arrest in children.

Several common medical conditions also can lead to breathing emergencies and cardiac arrest. For example, asthma, diabetes, seizures, and serious infections such as pneumonia can cause emergencies if they are not treated or controlled properly. Children with heart conditions,

Learning Objectives

After reading this chapter you will be able to

1. Name the links in the AHA pediatric Chain of Survival and discuss the role you play in the chain

2. Name the most common cause of death in infants from birth to 6 months of age

3. Describe the sleeping positions that reduce the risk of sudden infant death syndrome (SIDS)

4. List at least 3 of the 5 most common causes of fatal injury in infants and children

5. Describe how to safely restrain children up to 12 years old in a car

6. Describe ways to prevent injuries indoors and outdoors

7. List at least 2 signs of breathing emergencies in infants and children

8. Recognize breathing difficulty with poor air exchange, severe or complete foreign-body airway obstruction, respiratory arrest, and cardiac arrest in infants and children

respiratory (breathing) problems, or other chronic diseases have a higher risk of cardiac arrest and serious illness requiring emergency care.

If you know *when* to phone the emergency response number (or 911) and *how* to provide rescue breathing, chest compressions, and relief of foreign-body airway obstruction (FBAO), you can save a child's life.

The AHA pediatric Chain of Survival symbol (Figure 1) depicts the critical actions required to prevent and treat many life-threatening emergencies in infants and children, including cardiac arrest, respiratory arrest, and FBAO (choking). The pediatric Chain of Survival is a series of actions that link infants and children to the help they need. As the person responsible for the first links in the Chain of Survival, *you* link the infant or child victim to the best chance of survival in the community or the medical setting.

Cardiac arrest in infants and children is different from cardiac arrest in adults. *Sudden* cardiac arrest is much less common in infants and children than in adults. In adults cardiac arrest is usually caused by ventricular fibrillation (VF), an abnormal heart rhythm. In infants and children, cardiac arrest is usually the result of noncardiac causes such as SIDS or injuries. Because of these differences, the Chain of Survival for infants and children is different from the Chain of Survival for adults. This means that the order of actions you take for infants and children will differ from the order for adults.

Among people less than 21 years old, cardiac arrest occurs most commonly in infants (birth to 1 year old) and older adolescents. In the newly born (immediately after birth), respiratory failure is the most common cause of cardiac and breathing emergencies and cardiac arrest. In infants the most common cause of cause of death is SIDS. Other causes of cardiac and respiratory emergencies and cardiac arrest include respiratory diseases, airway obstruction (including FBAO), drowning, and severe infection. In children more than 1 year old, adolescents, and young adults, injuries are the leading cause of death.

In infants and children cardiac arrest typically develops as a complication of breathing difficulty or shock. Rescuers must recognize the early signs of breathing and cardiac problems in infants and children and intervene promptly to prevent cardiac arrest. Early CPR will significantly increase a child's chance of survival. Everyone who cares for children, including parents, childcare providers, teachers, and sports supervisors, should learn BLS. Parents of and childcare providers for children with conditions that increase their risk of cardiopulmonary failure or sudden cardiac arrest especially must learn BLS.

Response to Cardiovascular Emergencies in Infants and Children

Definitions of *Newly Born, Neonate, Infant, Child,* and *Adult*

A *neonate* is an infant up to 28 days (1 month) old. *Newly born* refers to a neonate up to a few *hours* old. The terms *newborn* and *neonate* were previously used to refer to the period immediately after birth, but those terms did not clearly distinguish between neonates within the first hours of life and those who were several days or weeks old. This distinction is important because advanced life support (ALS) is different for neonates and the newly born.

An *infant* is a child up to 1 year (12 months) old.

A *child* is 1 to 8 years old. For the purposes of BLS only, an *adult* is 8 years old or older.

Pediatric ALS includes infants, children, and adolescents.

For the purposes of BLS the term *infant* is defined by the approximate size of the young child who can be given effective chest compressions with 2 fingers or 2 thumbs (the rescuer's hands encircle the infant — these techniques are described in Chapter 5). To simplify BLS education, use of the term *child* in emergency cardiovascular care materials historically has been limited to victims between the ages of 1 and 8 years. Compressions can generally be given with 1 hand for victims 1 to 8 years old. But the size of the victim or the size and strength of the rescuer may require use of a different technique. For example, for a small toddler you may need to use the

---

FIGURE 1. The AHA pediatric Chain of Survival. The 4 links or sets of actions in the chain are **(1)** prevention of cardiac arrest and injuries, **(2)** early CPR, **(3)** early access to the emergency response system, and **(4)** early advanced care.

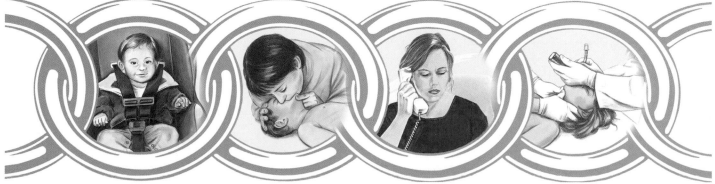

FYI: "Phone First" for Adults but "Phone Fast" for Infants and Children

Why a Lone Rescuer Should "Phone First" for an Unresponsive Adult Victim but "Phone Fast" After 1 Minute of CPR for an Unresponsive Pediatric Victim

When the initial ECG is obtained, most adults with sudden, nontraumatic cardiac arrest but no injuries are in VF. *For these victims the time from collapse to defibrillation is the greatest determinant of survival.* Defibrillation must be performed quickly. When no CPR is provided, survival from VF cardiac arrest falls by 7% to 10% for each minute without defibrillation. After 12 minutes of untreated VF cardiac arrest survival is unlikely, particularly if CPR is not provided. Phoning 911 (or other emergency response number) increases the victim's chance of survival because it shortens the time to defibrillation. If you find an un-responsive adult, activate the emergency response system (or phone 911). Your quick response will speed the arrival of emergency personnel with a defibrillator.

In infants (less than 1 year old) and children (1 to 8 years old), cardiopulmonary arrest is usually preceded by *airway* or *breathing* problems. In these victims *rescue support (especially rescue breathing)* is essential. Give rescue breaths and other resuscitation as needed for 1 minute and then call 911. This contribution of respiratory deterioration in the evolution of cardiopulmonary arrest in children provides the rationale for the "phone fast" approach to resuscitation in children.

Exceptions to the phone first/phone fast rule for adults and children include the following special situations:

1. **Near-drowning:** Provide 1 minute of rescue support (especially rescue breathing) for *all* victims of near-drowning and then phone 911.

2. **Cardiac arrest associated with injury:** Breathing problems may be present in injured victims. Provide 1 minute of rescue support (especially rescue breathing) for *all* victims of severe injury and then phone 911.

3. **Drug overdose:** Respiratory arrest or breathing problems often develop in victims of drug overdose. Provide 1 minute of rescue support (especially rescue breathing) for *all* victims of drug overdose and then phone 911.

4. **Children at risk for sudden cardiac arrest:** VF may be present in these victims. The lone rescuer should still give 1 minute of CPR and then phone the EMS system. If the child is 1 to 8 years of age, an AED may be used.

These exceptions are discussed in more detail in Chapter 6 of this manual. These instructions apply when you are the only rescuer present with the victim (for example, the lone rescuer). If a *second* rescuer is present, send that rescuer to phone 911 while you begin CPR. Healthcare providers will rarely find themselves performing resuscitation alone, so the 2-rescuer scenario is far more common than a "lone rescuer" scenario.

2-finger or 2-thumb technique. For a large 6- to 7-year-old child, you may need to use the 2-handed (adult) technique.

Anatomic and Physiologic Differences Affecting Cardiac Arrest and Resuscitation

Respiratory failure (breathing difficulties) or respiratory arrest frequently precedes cardiac arrest in infants and children. For this reason rescue breathing is emphasized in BLS for pediatric victims. For pediatric victims the lone rescuer opens the airway and gives rescue breaths before phoning 911. Remember, for pediatric victims provide CPR *first* and then phone the emergency response number.

For many reasons infants and children are at risk for airway problems that can lead to decreased oxygenation and cardiac arrest. The airway of an infant or child is smaller than the airway of an adult. Infants and children also have less oxygen reserve than adults. For these and

many other reasons, if breathing problems develop, infants and children can deteriorate rapidly. So support of breathing and oxygenation is extremely important for infants and children.

Cardiac output and systemic perfusion (blood flow) depends on an adequate heart rate. Bradycardia (a heart rate that is too slow) often develops just before cardiac arrest in infants and children. A major cause of bradycardia is hypoxia (lack of oxygen) caused by breathing difficulties or respiratory arrest. If bradycardia develops in an infant or child, immediately assess and support airway, breathing, and oxygenation. If the infant or child has a heart rate less than 60 beats per minute and signs of poor circulation (decreased responsiveness, cool extremities, weak pulse, and poor color) despite adequate airway, oxygenation, and ventilation, begin chest compressions.

Epidemiology of Cardiopulmonary Arrest: "Phone Fast" (Infant, Child)/ "Phone First" (Adult)

In *adults* sudden cardiopulmonary arrest is most often *cardiac* in origin. The most common heart rhythm is VF. For adults with VF the time from collapse to defibrillation is the greatest determinant of survival. Early CPR doubles the chance of survival after witnessed sudden cardiac arrest in adults.

Cardiac arrest in infants and children has many different causes. SIDS, near-drowning, injuries, and infection are some of the most common. These causes often produce respiratory failure or arrest before cardiac arrest. That is, they lead to breathing difficulties, and the breathing difficulties lead to hypoxemia, bradycardia, and cardiac arrest.

In the pediatric age group resuscitation is most frequently needed at the time of birth. About 5% to 10% of newly born infants require some degree of resuscitation at birth, including stimulation to breathe. About 1% to 10% of newly born infants delivered in the hospital require assisted breathing. Worldwide more than 5 million neonates die each year. Breathing difficulties at birth are responsible for nearly 1 million of these deaths. Use of relatively simple resuscitation techniques at birth could save an estimated 1 million infants per year.

Most out-of-hospital cardiac arrests in infants and children occur in or around the home, where children are under the supervision of parents or childcare providers. SIDS, injuries, drowning, poisoning, choking, severe asthma, and pneumonia are the most common causes of childhood arrest. In the United States and many other countries, injury is the leading cause of death from the age of 6 months through young adulthood.

The condition that precedes most out-of-hospital cardiac arrests in infants and children is breathing difficulty. Breathing difficulty progresses from hypoxia with bradycardia to cardiac arrest. That is, the heart rate slows and then the heart stops. Asystole (cardiac standstill) is present in most pediatric victims of cardiac arrest when EMS personnel arrive. Ventricular tachycardia (VT) or VF is less common in infants and children than in adult victims of cardiac arrest. However, infants and children with VT and VF often have a better chance of survival than those with asystole.

Immediate rescue breathing and chest compressions can restore circulation and increase the chance of survival in infants and children with cardiac arrest. Early defibrillation can improve outcome in children with VT or VF. Because cardiopulmonary arrest in infants and children is generally respiratory in origin, you should begin CPR

first (and phone later, that is, "phone fast") when you find an unresponsive infant or child outside the hospital. This approach is different from the approach to BLS for adult victims of cardiac arrest. In adults you "phone first" and *then* begin CPR and provide defibrillation (see FYI: "Phone First" for Adults but "Phone Fast" for Infants and Children).

BLS for Children With Special Needs

Children with chronic physical, developmental, behavioral, or emotional conditions have special healthcare needs. These children often require more (or different kinds of) healthcare services than typically developing children. Children with chronic conditions sometimes need emergency care for life-threatening complications related to their conditions. For example, a child with a tracheostoma (a surgically made opening in the windpipe used for breathing) may have an obstruction in the opening that is causing breathing difficulty.

Nonetheless, about half of all calls to EMS systems for children with special healthcare needs are unrelated to the child's special needs. Instead the calls are prompted by traditional causes of emergencies in children, such as injury. These emergencies require no special treatment beyond the normal EMS standard of care.

Emergency care of children with special healthcare needs can be complicated by lack of specific medical information about the child's condition, medical plan of care, current medications, and any "do not attempt to resuscitate" orders. The best source of information about a chronically ill child is the person who cares for the child on a daily basis. If that person is unavailable or unable to provide information (such as after a car crash), emergency personnel will need some means of obtaining important information.

A wide variety of methods have been developed to make such information immediately accessible. For example, standard forms, containers kept in a standard place in the home (such as the refrigerator), window stickers, wallet cards, and medical alert bracelets are some of the methods now used. No single method of communicating information has proved to be superior to the others. The American Academy of Pediatrics and the American College of Emergency Physicians developed the Emergency Information Form (EIF) for this purpose. This form is available through the Internet at www.pediatrics.org/cgi/content/full/104/4/e53.

If your child has special healthcare needs, keep essential medical information at home, with the child, and at the child's school or childcare facility. If you are a childcare provider, make sure you have access to this information (including any advance directives) and learn the signs of deterioration in the child.

If the physician, parents, and child (as appropriate) have decided to limit resuscitative efforts or to withhold attempts at resuscitation, the physician's order indicating the limits of resuscitative efforts must be written for use in the hospital. In most countries a separate order must be written for limitation of resuscitative efforts outside the hospital. Legal requirements for out-of-hospital no-CPR directives vary from country to country. In the United States the requirements vary from state to state. Families must inform the local EMS system when advanced directives are established for out-of-hospital pediatric or adult care.

Whenever a child with a chronic or life-threatening condition is discharged from the hospital, parents, school nurses, and any home healthcare providers should be informed about possible complications that the child may experience and anticipated signs of deterioration and their causes. Specific instructions should be given regarding CPR and other interventions that the child may require, as well as instructions about whom to contact and why.

If the child has a tracheostoma, teach everyone responsible for the child's care (including parents, school nurses, and home healthcare providers) how to determine if the airway is open, to clear the airway, and to provide CPR. Rescue breathing and bag-mask ventilation are performed through the tracheostomy tube in these children. As with any form of rescue breathing, you will know that rescue breaths are effective because the chest will rise. If the tracheostomy tube becomes obstructed, try to clear it with suctioning. If the tube still cannot be used, replace it. If a clean tube is not available, provide rescue breaths through the opening on the neck until an artificial airway can be inserted. If the upper airway is open, you may be able to provide effective breaths through the nose and mouth using a bag-mask device. To provide rescue breathing this way, you will need to block the opening on the neck so that air will not escape.

Out-of-Hospital (EMS) Care

EMS systems were initially created for adults. EMS equipment, training, experience, and expertise are less well developed to meet the needs of children. In the United States the death rate for children treated in EMS systems is higher than the death rate for adults treated in EMS systems, especially in areas where pediatric ALS is unavailable. To improve out-of-hospital care for infants and children, EMS personnel must be trained and equipped to care for pediatric victims, medical dispatchers must use emergency protocols appropriate for children, and Emergency Departments caring for children must be appropriately staffed and equipped. Emergency Departments that care for acutely ill or injured children should have an ongoing agreement with a tertiary care center through which patients can receive postresuscitation care in a pediatric intensive care unit under the supervision of trained personnel.

Reducing the Risk of SIDS, Injury, and Arrest

Healthcare providers are often able to teach parents and children about risk factors for injury and cardiac arrest. This section provides information about prevention of SIDS and injuries, the leading causes of death in infants and children. The appendix at the end of this chapter contains a safety checklist. Give this checklist to children and parents who visit your healthcare facility and suggest that they use it to identify ways to reduce childhood injuries and SIDS in and around the home. Use it to keep your own family safe, too.

Reducing the Risk of SIDS

SIDS is the sudden death of an infant that cannot be explained even after an autopsy. SIDS typically occurs in infants 1 month to 1 year old. The syndrome is probably caused by a variety of conditions and mechanisms that all result in death during sleep. For example, suffocation may occur if an infant rebreathes exhaled air while lying face down. Most SIDS deaths occur in the first 6 months of life. The highest number of deaths occur in infants 2 to 4 months old. Many factors are associated with an increased risk of SIDS: a prone sleeping position (on the stomach), the winter months, low family income, male gender, being a sibling of a SIDS victim, a mother who smokes or is addicted to drugs, a history of severe life-threatening events, and low birthweight.

Critical Concepts: Reduce Risk of SIDS: Avoid Prone Sleeping Position

To reduce the risk of SIDS, place healthy infants supine (on the back) to sleep.

- *Do not* place healthy infants prone (on the stomach) to sleep.

- Prop and position infants placed on their side to prevent them from rolling onto their stomachs.

- Do not place infants to sleep on soft materials such as a fluffy comforter or lamb's wool blanket.

Several years ago researchers discovered that SIDS occurred much more frequently among infants who slept on their stomach than among infants who slept on their back or side. Australia, New Zealand, and several European countries documented a significant decline in SIDS after parents and childcare providers were taught to place healthy infants on their back or side to sleep.

A "Back to Sleep" public education campaign began in the United States in 1992. That year approximately 7000 infants in the United States died of SIDS. In 1997, 5 years after the start of the campaign, only 2991 infants died of SIDS.

Anyone who cares for an infant must know to lay healthy infants on their back (supine position) to sleep. The supine sleeping position has not been associated with an increase in problems such as vomiting or aspiration. You may lay infants on their side, but position and support them so that they *cannot* roll onto their stomach.

Do not lay infants on or wrap them in soft materials such as a lamb's wool blanket or fluffy comforter. Do not allow infants to sleep with objects such as stuffed animals that might trap exhaled air near the face.

Injury: The Magnitude of the Problem

In the United States injuries are the leading cause of death in people aged 1 to 44 years. Injuries are responsible for more childhood deaths than all other causes combined. Internationally injury death rates are highest for children 1 to 14 years old and young adults 15 to 24 years old. The term *injury* is used as the cause of death rather than the term *accident* because injuries are often *preventable*. The term *accident* implies that nothing could have been done to prevent the event.

Causes and Prevention of Common Childhood and Adolescent Injuries

Injury prevention will have the greatest effect by focusing on injuries that are frequent and for which effective strategies are available. The leading causes of death internationally in children 1 to 14 years old are shown in Figure 2.

The 6 most common causes of fatal injury in children *that can be prevented* are motor vehicle passenger injuries, pedestrian injuries, bicycle injuries, submersion, burns, and firearm injuries. Prevention of these injuries would substantially reduce childhood deaths and disability. For this reason information about injury prevention is included with information about infant and child resuscitation.

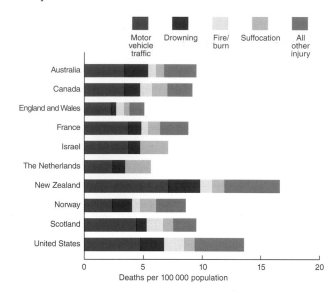

FIGURE 2. International rates of death due to injury in children 1 to 14 years old.

Motor Vehicle and Traffic Safety

Passenger Injuries

Injuries sustained while riding in a car are the No. 1 preventable cause of death in young children.

A young child is very "top heavy," and a young child's hips are difficult to anchor with a lap belt. For these reasons you must restrain young children in safety seats that secure the torso and the hips. Children who are not restrained tend to fly headfirst through the car when a collision occurs. Even in a low-speed crash an infant or small child can smash into the windshield, dashboard, or air bag with a force comparable to that of falling from a third-story window. Holding a child on your lap is *not* safe. If a crash occurs, the child will be thrown into the dashboard or crushed by your weight.

The BACK seat is the BEST seat for children *through 12 years of age.* A child who is properly restrained in the back seat is *least* likely to sustain injuries in a crash because the child is away from the dashboard, windshield, and front-seat air bags.

You have probably heard about injuries resulting from air bags. Air bags save lives when used with seat belts, and they can protect drivers and passengers who are correctly "buckled up." Air bags have saved more than 3000 lives nationwide since they were introduced. But air bags have fatally injured several children and even small adults. An air bag inflates quickly and forcefully to cushion a victim during a crash. During inflation an air bag can strike anything or anyone near the dashboard. The air bag inflates rapidly, with a great deal of force. Serious head

Critical Concepts:
Automobile Passenger Safety

- EVERYONE in the car must "buckle up" with age-appropriate restraint devices.
- The BEST seat is the BACK seat for children 12 years old and younger.
  - → **Never** place an infant in the front seat of a car with a passenger-side air bag.
  - → **Never** place a child in a child safety seat in the front seat of a car.
  - → Use proper child restraint devices (including belt-positioning booster seats) for children less than 4 feet 10 inches (less than 58 inches or less than 148 cm) tall and weighing less than 80 pounds (less than 36 kg).
  - → Use lap and shoulder belts for children at least 4 feet 10 inches (at least 58 inches or 148 cm) tall and weighing at least 80 pounds (at least 36 kg).
  - → Allow only adults and children more than 12 years old to sit in the front seat.
  - → Fatigue, medications, alcohol, and drugs can compromise a person's ability to drive.
- Never allow a child to ride in a vehicle with a driver who may be compromised by fatigue, medications, alcohol, or drugs. If you have any doubt about the driver's ability to drive, make other arrangements for your child's transportation.

and neck injuries and even death can result when passengers who are not properly restrained strike the air bag while it is inflating. Most of the people injured by air bags have *not* been properly restrained.

To prevent injuries caused by air bags, make sure everyone in the car is properly restrained. Do not allow young children (12 years old and younger) to ride in the front seat of the car. Do not place *any* car seat in the front seat. Car seats placed in the front seat position the child too close to the air bags. Rear-facing infant seats should not be placed in the front seat, because they will position the infant's head very close to the dashboard. If the air bag inflates, it will drive the infant seat into the passenger seat, injuring the infant's head and neck. The American Academy of Pediatrics, the Centers for Disease Control

and Prevention, and the National Highway Traffic Safety Administration recommend the following safety precautions:

- Use child restraint devices and lap and shoulder belts appropriate for the child's age and size.
- For infants weighing less than 20 pounds (less than 9 kg) and less than 1 year old:
  - → Use a rear-facing safety seat secured in the BACK seat of the car.
  - → *Never* place an infant in the front seat of a car with a passenger-side air bag.
  - → For children weighing more than 20 pounds (more than 9 kg) and 1 to 4 years old:
  - → Use a child safety seat secured in the BACK seat of the car.
- For children 4 through 12 years old:
  - → For children **less than 4 feet, 10 inches** (less than 58 inches or 148 cm) tall and **weighing less than 80 pounds** (less than 36 kg), use a belt-positioning booster seat secured in the BACK seat of the car.
  - → Children **at least 4 feet, 10 inches** (at least 58 inches or 148 cm) tall and **weighing at least 80 pounds** (at least 36 kg) can usually be properly restrained with both a lap and shoulder belt in the BACK seat of the car. Make sure the shoulder belt crosses the body from the shoulder, across the breastbone, down to the hip. Make sure the shoulder belt does *not* cross the face or neck. Make sure the lap belt fits snugly across the hips.
- For children more than 12 years old:
  - → Use lap and shoulder belts. Make sure the shoulder belt crosses the body from the shoulder, across the breastbone, down to the hip. Make sure it does not cross the face or neck.
  - → When children (or small adults) more than 12 years old are seated in the front seat, move the front seat as far away from the dashboard as possible.

When you secure a safety seat in a car, tighten the belt so that the seat does not move more than ½ inch (1 cm) in any direction. Push the seat forward, backward, and side to side to make sure it is secure.

For more information about children and air bags, call the National Highway Traffic Safety Administration Auto Safety Hotline (1-800-424-9393 or 1-888-327-4236) or visit their website (www.nhtsa.dot.gov).

Children learn by example. Be sure that you and every person who rides with you buckles up for *every* ride. Follow the watchwords of the American Academy of Pediatrics and "make every ride a safe ride." Remember: The BACK SEAT is the BEST SEAT for children 12 years old and younger.

Pedestrian and Bicycle Injuries

Not all children who die of injuries caused by motor vehicles are passengers in cars. Some are injured or killed while walking, playing near streets, or riding bicycles.

- Infant and toddler pedestrians are most commonly killed by cars backing out of driveways or parking lots.

- Children between the ages of 5 and 9 years old are most often injured when they dart out in front of traffic while playing or crossing the street in the middle of the block. Teach young children to cross streets at intersections, to always stop at curbs, and to *stop, look* both ways, and *listen* for cars before crossing any street.

- Children riding bicycles can be injured if they collide with cars or fixed objects or if they are thrown from the bicycle. *The most serious bicycle-related injuries are head injuries, which can cause death or permanent brain damage. The severity of bicycle-related head injuries can be reduced by about 85% if children wear bicycle helmets* approved by the Snell Memorial Foundation or the American National Standards Institute (ANSI) *every time* they ride a bicycle. The helmet must fit snugly to protect the child properly. For more information on selecting and using helmets, visit the American Academy of Pediatrics website at www.aap.org/family/thelmabt.htm.

Submersion or Drowning

Drowning is a major cause of death and disability in children. Drowning can occur indoors or outdoors. The bathtub is the most common site for drowning by infants up to 1 year old. Young children can drown in only a few inches of water. Always closely supervise infants, toddlers, and preschoolers in the bathtub or near any container of water, including buckets and toilets.

Keep toilet lids closed, and do not allow infants or toddlers to play near industrial-size buckets (5 gallons or larger) containing liquids. Young children have large, heavy heads. If they lean over and fall into a bucket or any large liquid container, their legs may be too light and their arms too weak to lift their head from the water.

Drowning in backyard swimming pools is a leading cause of death and permanent brain damage in children, particularly among children 1 to 4 years old. The natural curiosity of toddlers, their inability to understand the danger and depth of water, and the appeal of water play can be a dangerous combination. A young child is capable of getting into a swimming pool alone, but he may be incapable of getting out alone. **No child is "drown-proof."** The ability to swim does *not* prevent drowning.

Do not allow children to have unsupervised access to swimming pools. Completely surround all pools, hot tubs, and spas with a nonclimbable fence at least 5 feet high. Make sure the fence has a self-closing, self-latching gate. The house is not an adequate barrier to the pool because toddlers may leave the house and go to the pool area. Pool covers and alarms will not prevent drowning. A drowning child often sinks quietly without screaming for help or thrashing. If that happens, the child may never activate the pool alarm.

Always supervise children when they play in or around water. Remove all toys from the pool area after swimming so children will not be lured back into the water. Parents and older children who live in a home with a swimming pool should learn CPR.

Have children wear life vests when they play on docks, at beaches, or at rivers. Children who swim in moving water should wear approved flotation devices. *Do not allow any child to swim alone.*

Drowning in natural waters is a *relatively common cause of death in adolescent boys.* Closely supervising adolescents is difficult, but you can help prevent drowning by understanding why adolescents are at risk. Adolescents are risk-takers, and they are susceptible to peer pressure. These factors may cause adolescents to try to swim farther than they can or to swim in dangerous waters. Alcohol consumption may contribute to an adolescent's risk-taking behavior and lack of judgment.

Burns and Smoke Inhalation

Burns and smoke inhalation are common causes of death and injury in children, particularly young children. Most fire-related deaths and serious injuries are caused by smoke inhalation. *Smoke detectors are one of the most effective interventions to prevent death from burns and smoke inhalation in the home.* Install smoke detectors on each level of your home or childcare center, and keep them in working order.

Most smoke detectors require batteries. If the batteries are dead, the smoke detector will not work. Install new batteries in all smoke detectors *at least* every 6 months. If you think you might forget, change the batteries every fall and spring when you change the time on your clocks. Every home should have smoke detectors.

Develop and practice a fire evacuation plan for your home, and make sure your child's school or daycare center does the same. Practice evacuating the house or building several times each year. During practice make sure everyone can be evacuated and accounted for quickly.

Keep matches away from children, and do not smoke in bed. Electrical short circuits also may cause house fires and deaths. Do not use appliances with frayed cords or damaged plugs.

Most scalds in infants and children are caused when a hot liquid spills on the child. This burn injury is usually not fatal, but it can cause long-term disability. Scalds usually occur in the kitchen or bathtub. To prevent scald injuries, take the following precautions:

■ Kitchen: Toddlers often grab pot handles that extend over the edge of the stove, spilling the boiling contents on themselves. To prevent these injuries, turn pot handles toward the center and back of the stove.

■ Bathtub: Young children may turn on the hot water and be scalded. Water at a temperature of 140°F (60°C) causes a scald in 6 seconds; water at 120°F (48.9°C) must be in contact with the skin for about 5 minutes to cause a scald. To prevent scald injuries in the bathtub, check the temperature of your water heater. Make sure it is set between 120°F and 130°F (48.9°C and 54.4°C). Some water heaters are preset at 150°F.

Burns also can occur when a child comes into contact with a hot iron, a curling iron, or a heating source such as a wood stove or wall heater. These burns can be prevented. Keep irons out of your child's reach, and place a barrier around wood stoves, radiators, and other heating sources. Keep curtains, linens, and furniture well away from heaters.

Provide ventilation for kerosene and gasoline-powered heaters. Do not use these heaters in a closed space or closed room because carbon monoxide poisoning can develop.

Firearm Injuries

Injuries caused by firearms are a leading cause of death and disability in children, adolescents, and young adults. Although the number of these injuries has declined in recent years, firearm injuries are the leading cause of death among African American adolescents and young adults and the second-highest cause of death among all adolescents and young adults in the United States. These injuries may be unintentional or intentional (suicide or homicide).

Most firearm injuries result from handguns, and most child-related shootings involve guns from the home of the child victim or a friend. Guns in the home are often loaded, and they are often readily accessible to children (for example, under a pillow or in a drawer).

If you keep a gun in your home, ensure that the gun cannot be operated by unsupervised children. Store the gun *unloaded* and *locked*. Secure all firearms in a locked cabinet or drawer or lock box and use trigger locks on every one. Store the ammunition in a separate location. Check the guns daily to ensure that no one has touched them, played with them, or taken them.

Foundation Facts:
Safety Supplies for Areas Where Children Live and Play

■ **Emergency telephone numbers.** Post emergency numbers by the phone for quick reference.

■ **Smoke detector with a working battery.** Mount smoke detectors on the ceiling outside rooms where children play and sleep.

■ **Trigger locks or lock boxes for firearms.**

■ **Plastic plug covers for electric outlets.** Plug covers will protect children from electric shock.

■ **Plastic outlet covers.** Use outlet covers when an electric cord is plugged into the outlet. These covers will keep children from pulling the cord from the outlet.

■ **Cabinet latches and locks.** Install latches and locks on any cabinet or drawer where dangerous items such as medicines, cleaning products, and knives are stored.

■ **Hot water gauge** (such as a meat or candy thermometer). Measure the temperature of tap and bath water to prevent scalding.

■ **Door hook-and-eye latches.** Install latches on the doors to the basement, garage, or any area where dangerous products are stored. Be sure to install the latches well out of the reach of children.

These safety devices will help you reduce injuries and give you the satisfaction of knowing that you have taken steps to improve the safety of a child's environment.

Poisoning

Poisoning is common in children. More than 250,000 household products are available today, and many contain harmful chemicals. A wide variety of drugs are stored in the average home. These drugs are often stored in desk drawers and night stands, and they are readily accessible to children. It is not surprising that children, who are curious about everything, are often victims of poisoning.

Common poisons found in the home include

■ Prescription and nonprescription medications, particularly iron pills, vitamins containing iron, acetaminophen (such as Tylenol), and aspirin

■ Plants

■ Cleansers, polishing agents, ammonia, and detergents

■ Cosmetics and hair care products (such as hair-coloring agents)

■ Alcohol and liquor

■ Insect and rodent poisons and moth balls

■ Gasoline, kerosene, and other petroleum products

■ Pesticides, weed killers, and fertilizers

■ Lye and acids

■ Paint and paint thinners

The best place to obtain information about poisons is your regional poison control center. The staff can quickly provide accurate and up-to-date information about almost any poisonous or potentially poisonous product. They will also provide immediate first aid instructions and treatment recommendations. This service is available 24 hours a day. Write the telephone number of the nearest poison control center on a sticker, and post the sticker on or near the telephone. In an emergency phone 911.

In the past syrup of ipecac (a substance that causes vomiting) was recommended to reduce absorption of ingested poisons. But recent research has shown that syrup of ipecac is often *not* helpful, particularly if the child can reach medical care within 15 minutes. Inducing vomiting may even be harmful after ingestion of some toxic substances. *Always* check with the poison control center or your child's physician *before* giving syrup of ipecac.

To prevent poisoning, store medicines, vitamins, and household cleaning products in areas inaccessible to small children. *Never store poisons in empty food or drink containers.* For example, do *not* store kerosene in soda bottles. Buy containers designed for storing poisons and clearly label them. Store these containers well out of a child's sight and reach. A *high, locked cabinet* is the best place to store poisons. Locking up poisons is important. Resourceful children can stack objects and climb to reach toxic items stored on high shelves.

Check prescription and over-the-counter medications at least once a year. Flush all medications that are past their expiration date down the toilet. Do not throw expired or unneeded medications in a garbage can. Young children may find them.

Choking, Strangulation, and Suffocation

Choking and suffocation are among the most common causes of preventable death in children less than 1 year old. Choking and suffocation also cause many deaths in children up to 14 years old. Choking occurs when food, toys, or other objects block the windpipe (trachea). Strangulation is caused by constriction around the neck. Suffocation occurs when the nose, mouth, or windpipe is blocked.

The most common objects that cause **choking** in infants and children are

■ Foods such as hot dogs, grapes, nuts, popcorn, and hard candy

■ Toys or parts of toys that are small enough to place in the mouth; *do not allow infants and children to play with a toy that can fit through the tube of a roll of toilet paper*

■ Uninflated balloons or pieces of a burst balloon (these are particularly hard to remove from an infant's airway)

Critical Concepts:
Red Flags of a Breathing Emergency With Poor Air Exchange — Signs to Phone the Emergency Response Number

✔ Weak cry

✔ Inability to speak or a weak voice

✔ Decreasing alertness or responsiveness

✔ Blue or pale lips and inside of the mouth

✔ Very rapid breathing with evidence that the infant or child is working hard to breathe **or** very slow, shallow breathing (infant or child is barely breathing)

TABLE. Injury Prevention Strategies for Parents, Prospective Parents, Childcare Providers, Teachers, and Children

Cause of Injury	Steps to Prevent Injury
Motor vehicle crash	■ "Buckle up" EVERY passenger in the vehicle. ■ Children up to 4 years and weighing up to 40 lb (18 kg): Use child restraint devices. Be sure they are installed and secured correctly! ■ Children 40 to 80 lb (18 to 36 kg) and less than 4 feet, 10 inches (58 inches or 148 cm): Use a belt-positioning booster seat. ■ Children must be at least 58 in (148 cm) and at least 80 lb (36 kg) to be safely restrained in lap and shoulder belts alone. ■ Children 12 years or less should sit in the BACK seat.
Pedestrian struck by vehicle	■ Supervise children playing near driveways, streets, or traffic. ■ Teach children to *stop, look,* and *listen* before crossing the street and to use crosswalks.
Bicycle crash	■ Be sure all bike riders ALWAYS wear bicycle helmets (ANSI or Snell approved).
Drowning	■ Supervise children who are near water (including bathtubs and swimming pools) at all times. ■ Be sure that home swimming pools are completely surrounded by fences. ■ Be sure that children wear life vests when boating.
Firearms	■ Store all firearms UNLOADED and LOCKED.
Burns and smoke inhalation	■ Install smoke alarms. Change batteries at least twice a year (spring and fall). ■ Keep drapes and furniture away from heaters.
Poisoning	■ Keep all poisons out of the reach of children. ■ Do not store poisons in containers intended for drinking (for example, soft drink bottles). ■ Post the number of the poison control center near the phone.
SIDS, choking, and suffocation	■ Place healthy infants to sleep on their back or side. Do not place infants on their stomach to sleep. ■ Do not allow infants and small children to play with toys that are small enough to fit through the tube of a roll of toilet paper. ■ Do not allow children to play with plastic bags.
Falls	■ Place gates on all windows above the ground floor in rooms occupied by children. ■ Use gates to block stairways from infants and toddlers.

- Other small items such as coins, marbles, buttons, beads, watch or camera batteries, and safety pins

Strangulation of infants and children in the home is most often linked to

- Drapery and extension cords (tie cords well above the floor to keep them out of the reach of small children; eliminate loops of cord within the child's reach)

- Cords from which toys and objects such as rattles, pacifiers, and jewelry are hung around the child's neck

Suffocation in the home is linked to

- Plastic bags (carefully dispose of or store all plastic bags so that children cannot find them)

- Laying infants on their stomach to sleep (SIDS is less likely to occur if infants are laid on their back to sleep; do not lay infants on soft materials such as a lamb's wool blanket or a fluffy comforter or against stuffed animals)

Falls

Falls are commonplace and often minor in children. About 200 children die each year as a result of falls, but falls are the most frequent cause of nonfatal injury in children less than 6 years old. Infants and children may be injured by

- Falls out of sinks or bathtubs or off countertops or changing tables

- Climbing out of a crib

- Falls down stairs. Twenty percent of all falls occur on stairs. Keep stairways as safe as possible. Provide adequate lighting, remove toys, tack down loose carpet, and use appropriate gate enclosures. Do not use accordion-type gates with wide gaps at the top. Instead use a safety gate that is permanently mounted or firmly attached to the wall with double closures that cannot be operated by children.

- Falls associated with infant walkers, especially near stairs or ramps

- Falls from upper-floor windows. Open windows only from the top or 4 to 5 inches from the bottom. Secure windows at the proper height with a burglar lock (available at hardware stores). Place gates over the lower portion of windows in high-rise buildings.

- Falls from trees or play equipment

Playground Injuries

Children are frequently injured at the playground. Although playground injuries are not often fatal, they are common and can require medical care or hospitalization. The number and severity of these injuries can be reduced if we ensure that all playground equipment is safe. Attachments, cables, and seats of swings should be inspected regularly, particularly at the beginning and middle of every summer, and they should be kept in good condition at all times. School playgrounds should be inspected before and during the middle of every school year. Playgrounds should be built on several (4 to 6) inches of an energy-absorbing surface such as sand, wood chips, or rubber padding. Concrete and grass do *not* provide adequate cushioning for children when they fall.

Safety Checklist

The injury prevention strategies in the Table and the safety checklist in the Appendix will help you make your child's daily environment as safe as possible. These strategies are based on the most up-to-date information on injury, and the checklist is designed to guide you through an inspection of your home, childcare center, school, babysitter's home, or wherever your children spend time.

Share this with parents of children whom you meet at work. Suggest that parents and childcare providers use it to inspect their home and childcare center. Tell them to note areas that need correction. You can help prevent injury and death of the children around you by following the recommendations in the course video and those listed in the checklist. See the Table and Foundation Facts: Safety Supplies for Areas Where Children Live and Play.

Signs of Breathing Emergencies and Cardiac Arrest in Infants and Children

How to Recognize Breathing Emergencies

In children breathing emergencies can lead to cardiac arrest. Breathing emergencies can be characterized by *increased* or *decreased* breathing effort. Foreign-body airway obstruction (FBAO), croup (a viral infection causing a hoarse cough), asthma, serious pneumonia, or drowning may cause *increased* breathing effort. A child with any of these conditions is struggling to breathe and may breathe very rapidly. The rescuer must decide whether the child's breathing is resulting in *poor* or *good* air exchange. Poor air exchange requires emergency treatment. Good air exchange provides sufficient air movement and does not require emergency treatment.

Signs of *poor* air exchange include a weak cry, inability to speak or a weak voice, decreasing alertness or responsiveness, and blue or pale lips and mucous membranes (inside the mouth, including the tongue). If you observe these signs, *phone the emergency response number* and make sure that the airway is open.

Children with a *decreased* breathing effort breathe very slowly or very shallowly, so they cannot maintain sufficient oxygen in the blood. If this condition is not corrected, it can lead to respiratory or cardiac arrest. Head injury, drug intoxication, and certain medical conditions can cause decreased breathing effort. Children with decreased breathing effort require rescue breathing and emergency treatment. Children who are deprived of oxygen may suffer a cardiac arrest.

Critical Concepts:
Signs of Severe or Complete Airway Obstruction

The following signs of severe or complete airway obstruction in a responsive infant or child require immediate action:

- **Universal sign of choking** (hands clutching the throat). The infant will not make this sign.

- Inability to speak. The infant will be unable to make loud sounds of any kind. Ask "Are you choking?" If the child nods yes, ask "Can you speak?" If the child shakes his head no or is unable to speak, severe or complete airway obstruction is present.

- Weak, ineffective coughs

- High-pitched sounds or no sounds while inhaling

- Increased difficulty breathing

- Bluish skin color (cyanosis)

You do *not* need to act if the child can cough forcefully or speak. Do not interfere at this point because a strong cough is the most effective way to remove a foreign body. Stay with the child and monitor her condition. If the partial obstruction persists, phone the emergency response number.

Signs of Severe or Complete FBAO (Choking)

Signs of severe or complete FBAO in infants and children include the *sudden* onset of weak or silent coughing, inability to speak, stridor (a high-pitched sound while inhaling or wheezing), and increased difficulty breathing. These signs may also be caused by *infections* such as epiglottitis and croup, which produce airway edema (swelling of the tissues in the airway). Signs of FBAO (rather than *infectious* airway obstruction) typically develop suddenly with no other signs of illness or infection, such as fever, signs of congestion, hoarseness, drooling, lethargy, or limpness.

If the child has an *infectious* cause of airway obstruction, signs of infection will be present. Back blows, chest thrusts, and abdominal thrusts will *not* relieve the obstruction. Immediately take the child to an emergency facility. If you think the signs of airway obstruction are caused by a foreign body, perform back blows and chest thrusts (for infants) or abdominal thrusts (for children). These techniques are described in Chapter 5.

Signs of Respiratory Arrest in Infants and Children

Respiratory arrest is present when the infant or child is not breathing at all or when breathing is clearly inadequate to maintain effective oxygenation and ventilation. The infant or child with respiratory arrest requires immediate support. You must open the airway and provide rescue breathing. These actions will prevent cardiac arrest and injury to the brain and other organs.

Respiratory arrest outside the hospital can result from a number of causes. For example, submersion or near-drowning, poisoning or drug overdose, lightning strike, smoke inhalation, respiratory infection, electrocution, suffocation, FBAO, head injuries, or coma may cause respiratory arrest. Inside the hospital drug reactions, sedation, increased intracranial pressure, or coma may cause respiratory arrest. When primary respiratory arrest occurs, the heart and lungs can continue to supply oxygen to the blood, brain, and other vital organs for several minutes. If you provide rescue breathing immediately, particularly with supplemental oxygen, delivery of oxygen to the brain and other vital organs may be maintained, and you may prevent the development of cardiac arrest.

Critical Concepts:
Red Flags of Cardiac Arrest

The 3 red flags of cardiac arrest are

1. No response
2. No adequate breathing
3. No signs of circulation — no adequate breathing, no coughing, no movement, no pulse

Signs of Cardiac Arrest

The infant or child who is in cardiac arrest will be unresponsive, will have no adequate breathing, and will have no signs of circulation (including no pulse). You will recognize cardiac arrest when you begin to provide BLS for the unresponsive infant or child. Open the airway and look, listen, and feel for breathing. If you find no adequate breathing, give 2 rescue breaths. The breaths should make the chest rise. Then check for signs of circulation, including a pulse. If no signs of circulation are present (see Critical Concepts: Red Flags of Cardiac Arrest), the child is in cardiac arrest. If you are in a healthcare facility, ECG monitoring can detect or confirm the development of an arrhythmia (VT or VF) consistent with cardiac arrest.

Cardiac arrest is often a sudden event in adults, but it does not often develop suddenly in infants or children. Cardiac arrest in infants and children most often develops as a complication of breathing difficulties, shock, or injuries (see Critical Concepts: Red Flags of Cardiac Arrest).

Remember: An unresponsive child may be in cardiac arrest. An unresponsive child is a red flag for an emergency: Act immediately!

Critical Concepts:
Causes of Cardiac Arrest — Differences Between Infants and Children and Adults

Infants and Children	Adults
■ Often caused by breathing emergencies	■ Usually caused by abnormal heart rhythm
■ Onset often follows illness or injury	■ Onset is often sudden
■ Primary heart rhythm problems are uncommon, especially in children less than 8 years old	■ Breathing emergencies are less common than sudden cardiac arrest

Learning Checklist

Review the key information you learned in this chapter.

- The 4 links in the AHA infant and child Chain of Survival are

  — Prevention of cardiac arrest and injuries

  — Early CPR

  — Early access to the emergency response system

  — Early advanced care

- The risk of SIDS can be reduced if infants are placed on their back or side to sleep.

- Injury due to motor vehicle crashes is the leading cause of death in infants and children. Many of these fatal injuries are preventable with relatively simple strategies:

  — All passengers must wear age-appropriate restraint devices

  — Proper restraint of children in the car is the most important preventive intervention.

  — The BACK seat is the BEST seat for children 12 years old or younger.

  — Never place an infant (rear-facing) safety seat in the front seat of a car.

  — Properly secure car seats following the manufacturer's installation instructions.

- Fatal bicycle injuries most often result from head injury.

  — Collisions with motor vehicles and falls from the bike cause serious injuries.

  — Bicycle helmets will prevent most bicycle-related head injuries.

- Drowning is the second most common cause of injury-related death in children 1 to 4 years old. Drowning occurs not only in pools and open bodies of water but also in bathtubs, toilets, or buckets. Always watch toddlers in the bathroom and make sure buckets are empty in areas where children live or play.

  — Drowning is most common in 2 age groups, toddlers (1 to 4 years old) and adolescent boys.

  — Pool covers and alarms are not foolproof. Surround pools with a fence on all sides, and make sure gates are self-closing and self-latching.

  — Adolescents have a higher risk of drowning because they like to take risks, they do not like to use safety equipment, and they will sometimes use alcohol or drugs while swimming or boating.

✔ Keep small objects away from children to reduce the risk of choking. Do not allow children to play and eat at the same time. Do not allow young children to play with toys that are small enough to fit through the tube of a toilet paper roll.

✔ Prevent burns and smoke inhalation by taking simple precautions.

— Mount smoke detectors on the ceiling outside bedrooms. Check smoke detectors monthly and replace batteries twice a year.

— Keep pots and other hot items out of the reach of toddlers.

— Set the temperature of your water heater at 120°F to 130°F (48.9°C to 54.4°C).

— Check electric cords for fraying, and cover all plugs and outlets.

✔ Store firearms locked, unloaded, and out of the reach of children.

✔ Keep medicines and household toxins out of the reach of children. Secure cabinets and drawers with childproof latches or locks.

✔ Signs of a breathing emergency with poor air exchange are

— Weak cry

— Inability to speak or a weak voice

— Decreasing responsiveness

— Blue or pale lips and mucous membranes (inside the mouth)

— Very rapid breathing with evidence that the child is working hard to breathe **or** very slow, shallow breathing (child is barely breathing)

✔ Signs of cardiac arrest in infants and children are

— No response

— No adequate breathing

— No signs of circulation (including no pulse)

Review Questions

1. You are driving your 9-month-old niece to the store. Where should you place her car seat in your vehicle?

   a. next to you

   b. in the rear center seat facing backward

   c. in the front seat facing forward

   d. in the front seat facing backward

2. What is the correct method of securing an infant car seat in the car?

   a. secure the car seat loosely so that the seat moves freely within the lap and shoulder belt

   b. keep the front seat close to the dashboard to prevent too much movement in a crash

   c. secure the car seat in the back seat so that it does not move

   d. secure the car seat using only the lap belt

3. You are in the process of trying to childproof your home. Which of the following statements is true about choking and strangling?

   a. choking and strangling do not cause death in children

   b. choking and strangling can be prevented by not allowing children to play with toys or objects that will fit through the center of a roll of toilet paper

   c. choking and strangling occur only in the home

   d. choking and strangling occur only during infancy and childhood

4. You are baby-sitting 2 young children by the local pool. Effective drowning prevention includes

   a. always watching children in or around water

   b. using water wings while swimming

   c. keeping life preservers in a locker on the boat

   d. letting a 5-year-old watch an infant in the bathtub

5. You have purchased a bicycle for your young son. The most effective device to reduce bicycle-related injuries is

   a. a safety helmet

   b. bike reflectors

   c. training wheels

   d. wrist and knee pads

6. You are trying to make your home safer, and you decide to post important emergency information on a sticker by the phone. Which of the following items do you *not* need to include?

   a. the telephone numbers for the EMS system, police, and fire department

   b. the telephone numbers for the local hospital and poison control center

   c. the social security number for each of your children

   d. your home telephone number

7. A 6-year-old who has come for a routine visit to the doctor collapses suddenly in your presence. What is the first action you perform for an unresponsive infant or child?

   a. phone the emergency response number

   b. shout for help and ask someone to phone the emergency response number and get the AED while you begin CPR

   c. perform rescue breathing and if there is no response, phone 911 and get the defibrillator

   d. transfer to advanced care

8. You are asked to talk to a Girl Scout troop about emergency cardiovascular care. You decide to use the Chain of Survival to illustrate the importance of preparation. What is the correct order of the links in `the AHA pediatric Chain of Survival?

   a. early access to the emergency response system, early CPR, early advanced care, prevention of injuries and arrest

   b. prevention of infection, early access to the emergency response number, early CPR, early advanced care

   c. early CPR, early activation of the emergency response system, prevention of injuries and arrest, early advanced care

   d. prevention of injuries and arrest, early CPR, early access to the emergency response system, early advanced care

9. You work in a daycare center and must decide when and when not to phone 911. Which of the following signs would most likely be caused by a breathing emergency and would require you to phone 911?

   a. child who is responsive but is very sleepy, is breathing rapidly and shallowly, and has blue skin or lips

   b. a loud, hoarse cough in an infant who is alert and smiling

   c. rapid breathing in a child who has a fever and is speaking normally

   d. deep, regular breaths in a child who is sound asleep

10. While visiting the cafeteria you see a 4-year-old girl who appears to be in distress. You suspect she may have a foreign-body airway obstruction. Which of the following signs indicate severe or complete FBAO in a child?

    a. the child can cough loudly and can speak

    b. the child is breathing quietly and has pink lips

    c. the child cannot speak, cry, or cough

    d. the child wheezes when she breathes in, but she can speak and cough

11. A 2-year-old-boy collapses in the waiting room of the doctors' office where you work. The child is unresponsive. You perform the assessment and support steps of CPR. Which of the following signs are the red flags of cardiac arrest?

    a. the child suddenly becomes unresponsive and his lips are blue

    b. the child stiffens and then has a seizure

    c. the child has no response, has no normal breathing, and no pulse or other signs of circulation

    d. the child has severe breathing difficulty and is unable to cry or speak

How did you do?

1, b; **2**, c; **3**, b; **4**, a; **5**, a; **6**, c; **7**, b; **8**, d; **9**, a; **10**, c; **11**, c.

Safety Checklist

This Safety Checklist was designed to help you make your home or work environment as safe as possible for infants and children. It can be used to inspect your home, the childcare center where your children stay after school, or any other place where children spend time. Take time to go around your house and see just how safe your home is for a child and learn how you can make it safer.

If you already follow the suggested safety precaution, check the box in the first column. If you need to purchase a certain item to make your home safer, the box on the far right will be shaded, indicating the need to purchase a "Safety Item." Check the shaded box when you have purchased the appropriate safety items.

	I follow this safety precaution (✔ = yes)	Purchase of safety item is required for all shaded boxes (✔ = item purchased)
Car Safety		
1. Ensure that every person in the car "buckles up" correctly.		
2. Have children less than 12 years old ride in the BACK seat with appropriate child restraints or lap-shoulder restraints.		
3. Use a rear-facing infant safety seat until infants weigh at least 20 lb and are 1 year old. ■ Secure all car seats in the BACK seat of the car. ■ Secure the seat following the manufacturer's instructions. ■ Test for tightness by pushing the seat forward, backward, and side to side. Tighten the belt to ensure that the seat does not move more than ½ inch (1 cm). ■ For proper adjustment, the seat belt buckle and latch plate (if needed) must be located well below the frame or toward the center of the seat.		☐ **Safety item — infant safety seat**
4. Wait until a child weighs 20 lb (9 kg) and is at least 1 year old and can sit with good head control before using a convertible seat or toddler seat in the forward-facing position. Place these seats in the BACK seat of the car.		☐ **Safety item — child safety seat**
5. Use a belt-positioning booster seat for children weighing 40 to 80 lb (18 to 36 kg). Secure the seat with a 3-point seat belt (lap and shoulder belt) in the BACK seat of the car. ■ If a shield is provided, fasten it close to the child's body. ■ Properly install the tether harness if required.		☐ **Safety item — belt-positioning booster seat**

	I follow this safety precaution (✔ = yes)	Purchase of safety item is required for all shaded boxes (✔ = item purchased)
Car Safety *(continued)*		
6. Children cannot be properly restrained with a lap-shoulder belt until they are at least 4 feet 9 inches (58 inches or 148 cm) tall, weigh 80 lb (36 kg), and can sit in the automobile seat with their knees bent over the edge. Always use a combination lap-shoulder belt to restrain children sitting in an automobile seat. ■ The shoulder belt should fit across the shoulder and breastbone. If it crosses the face and neck, use a belt-positioning booster seat to ensure that the belt is properly placed. Do not hook the shoulder belt under the child's arm. ■ All children 12 years old or younger should ride in the BACK seat.		
General Indoor Safety		
7. Place a sticker with emergency telephone numbers near or on the telephone. Include numbers for the EMS system, police, fire department, local hospital or physician, the poison control center in your area, and your telephone number.		☐ **Safety item — phone sticker with emergency response numbers**
8. Install smoke detectors on the ceiling in the hallway outside sleeping or napping areas and on each floor at the head of stairs. Test the alarm monthly and replace batteries twice a year (for example, in the fall and spring when the time changes to and from daylight saving time).		☐ **Safety item — smoke detector**
9. Ensure that there are 2 unobstructed emergency exits from the home, childcare center, classroom, or other facility where children are likely to be present.		
10. Develop and practice a fire escape plan.		
11. Ensure that a working fire extinguisher is on the premises.		☐ **Safety item — fire extinguisher**
12. All space heaters are approved; in safe condition; out of a child's reach; placed at least 3 feet from curtains, papers, and furniture; and have protective covers.		
13. All wood-burning stoves are inspected yearly and vented properly. Place stoves out of a child's reach.		

	I follow this safety precaution (✔ = yes)	Purchase of safety item is required for all shaded boxes (✔ = item purchased)
General Indoor Safety *(continued)*		
14. Ensure that electric cords are not frayed or overloaded. Place out of a child's reach.		
15. Install "shock stops" (plastic outlet plugs) or outlet covers on all electric outlets.		☐ **Safety item — plastic outlet plugs**
16. To prevent falls, always keep one hand on the infant while he or she is on a high surface such as a changing table.		
17. Position healthy full-term infants on their back or side to sleep. *Do not place infants on their stomach to sleep.*		
18. The crib is safe. ■ The crib mattress fits snugly with no more than 2 fingers' breadth between the mattress and crib railing. ■ The distance between crib slats is less than 2⅜ inches (so the infant's head won't get caught).		
19. Check the strength of stairs, railings, porches, and balconies.		
20. Light hallways and stairways to prevent falls.		
21. Use toddler gates at the top and bottom of stairs. (Do not use accordion-type gates with wide spaces at the top. They can entrap a child's head and cause strangulation.)		☐ **Safety item — toddler gates (NOT accordion-type)**
22. Do not let your child use an infant walker.		
23. To prevent falls, place locks (available at hardware stores) on all windows. Put gates on the lower part of open windows.		☐ **Safety item — window locks, gates**
24. Store medicines and vitamins out of a child's reach and in child-resistant containers.		☐ **Safety item — child-resistant containers**
25. Store cleaning products out of a child's reach and sight. ■ Store and label all household poisons in their original containers in high locked cabinets (not under sinks). ■ Do not store chemicals or poisons in soda bottles. ■ Store cleaning products separately from food.		

	I follow this safety precaution (✔ = yes)	Purchase of safety item is required for all shaded boxes (✔ = item purchased)
General Indoor Safety *(continued)*		
26. Install safety latches or locks on cabinets that contain potentially **dangerous items and are within a child's reach.**		☐ Safety item — safety latches or locks on cabinets
27. Keep purses containing vitamins, medications, cigarettes, matches, jewelry, and calculators (which have easy-to-swallow button batteries) out of a child's reach.		
28. Install a lock or hook-and-eye latch on the door leading to the basement or garage to prevent children from entering those areas. Place a lock at the top of the door frame.		☐ Safety item — latch on basement, garage doors
29. Keep potentially harmful plants out of a child's reach. (Many plants are poisonous. Consult your poison control center.)		
30. Be sure that toy chests have lightweight lids, no lids, or safe-closing hinges.		
Kitchen Safety		
31. To minimize the risk of burns: ■ Keep hot liquids, foods, and cooking utensils out of a child's reach. ■ Place hot liquids and food away from the edge of the table. ■ Cook on the back burners when possible and turn pot handles toward the center of the stove. ■ Avoid using tablecloths and place mats that can be yanked off, spilling hot liquids or food. ■ Keep high chairs and stools away from the stove. ■ Do not keep snacks near the stove. ■ Teach young children the meaning of the word *hot*.		
32. Keep all foods and small items (including balloons) that can choke a child out of reach. Test toys for size with a toilet-paper roll (if it fits inside the roll, it can choke a small child).		
33. Keep knives and other sharp objects out of a child's reach.		
Bathroom Safety		
34. Bathe children in no more than 1 or 2 inches of water. Stay with infants and young children throughout the bath.		

	I follow this safety precaution (✔ = yes)	Purchase of safety item is required for all shaded boxes (✔ = item purchased)
Bathroom Safety (*continued*)		
35. Use skidproof mats or stickers in the bathtub.		☐ Safety item — bath mats or stickers
36. Adjust the maximum temperature of the water heater to 120° to 130°F (48.9° to 54.4°C) or medium heat (test with a thermometer).		
37. Keep electrical appliances (radios, hair dryers, space heaters, etc) out of the bathroom or unplugged, away from water, and out of a child's reach.		
Firearms		
38. If firearms are stored in the home, they must be locked and inaccessible to children. Store guns individually locked and unloaded, and store ammunition separately.		☐ Safety item — trigger lock, lock-boxes for firearms
Outdoor Safety		
39. Playground equipment is assembled and anchored correctly according to manufacturer's instructions over a level, cushioned surface such as sand or wood chips.		
40. Your child knows the rules of safe bicycling. ■ Wear a protective helmet. ■ Use the correct size bicycle. ■ Ride on the right side of the road (*with* traffic). ■ Use hand signals and wear bright or reflective clothing.		☐ Safety item — bicycle helmet
41. Do not allow children to play with fireworks.		
42. Your child is properly protected while roller skating or skateboarding. ■ Child wears helmet and protective padding on knees and elbows. ■ Child skates only in rinks or parks that are free of traffic.		☐ Safety item — helmet and protective padding
43. Your child is properly protected while riding on sleds or snow disks. ■ Child sleds only in daylight and only in a safe, supervised area away from motor vehicles.		
44. Your child is properly protected while participating in contact sports. ■ Proper adult instruction and supervision are provided. ■ Teammates are of similar weight and size. ■ Appropriate safety equipment is used.		☐ Safety item — safety equipment for contact sports

	I follow this safety precaution (✔ = yes)	Purchase of safety item is required for all shaded boxes (✔ = item purchased)
Outdoor Safety *(continued)*		
45. To reduce the risk of animal bites: ■ Teach your child how to handle and care for a pet. ■ Teach your child never to try to separate fighting animals, even when a familiar pet is involved. ■ Teach your child to avoid unfamiliar animals.		
46. If you have a home swimming pool, be sure the pool is totally enclosed with fencing at least 5 feet high and that all gates are self-closing and self-latching. There should be no direct access (without a locked gate) from the home into the pool area. In addition ■ Children must *always* be supervised by an adult when swimming. Never allow a child to swim alone. ■ Change young children from swimsuits into street clothes and remove all toys from the pool area at the end of swim time. ■ All adults and older children should learn CPR. ■ Pools on nearby properties should be protected from use by unsupervised children.		**Safety item — 5-foot fence around swimming pool with self-closing, self-latching gate**

Note: Much of the safety information presented in this course is based on the SAFEHOME program developed by the Massachusetts Department of Public Health as part of its Statewide Comprehensive Injury Prevention Program and the Children's Traffic Safety Program at Vanderbilt University in Nashville, Tenn. The SAFEHOME program was funded by the Federal Division of Maternal and Child Health. The Children's Traffic Safety Program was funded by the Department of Transportation and the Tennessee Governor's Highway Safety Program.

You work in the Emergency Department of a hospital. A man rushes through the door and hands you a limp 3-year-old child. The child does not respond to your voice or touch, and his lips are blue. The man says, "He just went under in my pool 2 blocks from here. I got to him as fast as I could, but I had trouble finding him under the water. I don't know what to do. Can you help me?"

How would you assess the child? What would be your first action if the child did not respond?

You work in the Emergency Department of a hospital. A woman runs in with a limp infant in her arms. She yells for help. You take the infant and note immediately that he does not respond to your touch or voice. You shout for help and take the infant into the pediatric triage room and lay him down on a gurney.

The woman tells you that the infant, her son David, has had a high fever and has been fussy. While she was driving to the hospital, David had a seizure and stopped breathing. The infant is limp and his lips are dusky.

You grab a bag-mask device and turn on the oxygen. You open David's airway with a head tilt–chin lift, and you look, listen, and feel for breathing. The infant is gasping, so you give 2 breaths using the bag-mask device with 100% oxygen. His chest rises with each breath. After the second breath, he begins to cough and move. You feel a strong pulse. Your colleagues place ECG monitor leads on the infant's chest, and they establish IV access.

What type of arrest did David have? Why were your actions lifesaving? How would David's condition be different if you had not quickly provided rescue breathing?*

*Modified from *BLS for Healthcare Providers*, Chapter 9: Pediatric Basic Life Support.

The ABCs of CPR: Infant and Child CPR and Relief of Choking (FBAO)

CPR: The Second Link in the Chain of Survival for Infants and Children

Early CPR is the second link in the AHA infant/child Chain of Survival. CPR steps consist of *assessments* and the *skills* needed to support the airway, breathing, and circulation (Figure 1). CPR is performed in 3 basic steps known as the ABCs of CPR: **A**irway, **B**reathing, and **C**irculation. At each step you first must *assess* the victim and then provide the support the victim needs (that is, use the *skill*).

CPR helps to deliver oxygen to the blood and to move that oxygenated blood to the brain and other vital organs until medical treatment can restore normal heart action. Two primary CPR *skills* are rescue breathing or ventilation (blowing) and chest compressions (pumping).

If you find an *unresponsive* child, shout for help and begin CPR. If someone else is with you or responds to your shout, send that person to phone the emergency response number (or 911). Prevention of injuries and cardiac arrest, early CPR, and early access to the emer-

> ### Learning Objectives
>
> After reading this chapter you will be able to
>
> 1. Describe and demonstrate 1-rescuer and 2-rescuer CPR for an infant and child with and without a barrier device
>
> 2. Demonstrate rescue breathing with a bag-mask device
>
> 3. Describe and demonstrate how to clear the airway in a responsive and an unresponsive infant or child with complete foreign-body airway obstruction (FBAO)

gency response system are the first 3 links in the AHA pediatric Chain of Survival, and they are in your hands. If you are alone, perform CPR for 1 minute and then phone the emergency response number. The fourth link in the pediatric Chain of Survival, early advanced care, is provided by physicians, nurses, paramedics, and other healthcare providers with advanced training.

FIGURE 1. The steps of CPR for infants and children. CPR includes both assessment and support steps, performed in sequence. The rescuer provides only the support the victim needs.

Phone 911

Continue "pump and blow" for 1 minute

If no signs of circulation: begin chest compressions

Assess for signs of circulation

If no breathing: give 2 rescue breaths

If no response: open the airway: look, listen, and feel for breathing

Assess responsiveness

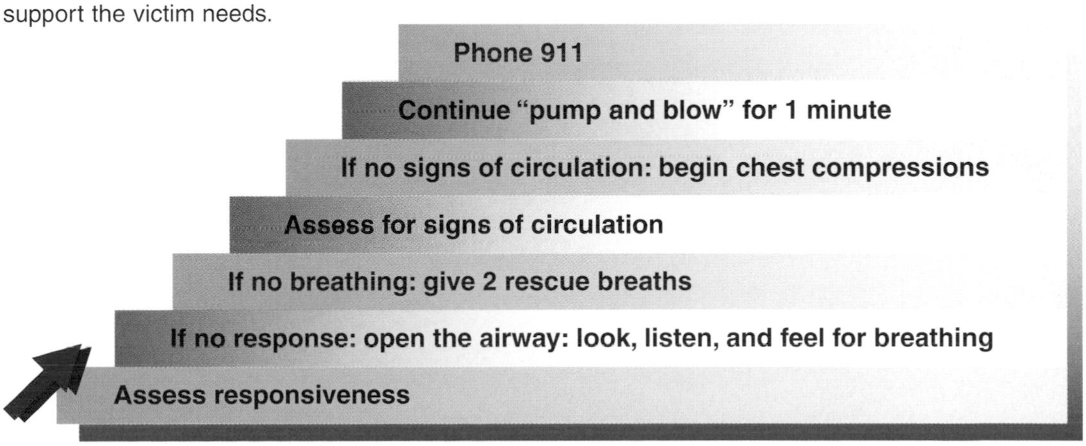

Critical Concepts:
Chain of Survival Sequence for Infants and Children With Heart Disease

Some infants or children with heart disease are at high risk for sudden cardiac arrest. If a child with known heart disease suddenly collapses, it may be best to follow the sequence of actions in the adult Chain of Survival rather than the pediatric Chain of Survival. If your child has heart disease, ask your child's physician or nurse which sequence to use. In the pediatric Chain of Survival, you *first perform CPR for 1 minute* and then phone 911 ("phone fast"). In the adult Chain of Survival, you *first phone 911* and then perform CPR ("phone first"). The adult Chain of Survival is described in Chapter 1 of this manual. CPR for adults is described in Chapter 2.

Heart disease and abnormal heart rhythms are the most common causes of sudden cardiac arrest in adults. But heart disease is a relatively *uncommon* cause of cardiac arrest in infants and children. The typical cause of cardiac arrest in infants and children is a lack of oxygen supply to the heart and brain caused by a breathing problem, respiratory arrest, or shock. Breathing emergencies can be caused by choking, suffocation, airway disease, lung disease, submersion or near-drowning, or injuries involving the airway or brain. If an infant or child stops breathing and no treatment is provided, cardiac arrest quickly follows. If you immediately provide rescue breathing for a victim with a breathing emergency, you may prevent cardiac arrest.

Critical Concepts:
CPR for Infants and Children

■ Check response.

■ If the child is unresponsive, shout for help.

■ Begin CPR.

Check response by shouting to the child. Gently tap the child's foot or arm. If the child does not respond, **shout for help.** Then begin **CPR.**

If other rescuers are present, send someone to phone the emergency response number (or 911).

Critical Concepts:
Opening the Airway

After you check responsiveness you open the airway. *Remember: The tongue is the most common cause of a blocked airway in an unresponsive victim.* When a victim is unresponsive, the muscles of the jaw and neck relax. When these muscles relax, the tongue falls back against the throat and blocks the airway (Figure 4A and 4B).

To open the airway, tilt the head back and lift the chin. This technique is called the *head tilt–chin lift.* The tongue is attached to the lower jaw. When you tilt the victim's head and lift the chin, you pull the victim's tongue away from the back of the throat. This action opens the victim's airway (Figure 2A and 2B).

If you think the victim has a head or neck injury, *do not* use the head tilt–chin lift. Instead use the *jaw thrust* to open the airway. To perform the jaw thrust, place one or more fingers under the angles of the victim's jaw. Lift the jaw forward *without* tilting the head. The jaw thrust pulls the tongue away from the back of the throat without excessively moving the head or neck (Figure 3). The jaw thrust is used only for victims with head and neck injuries because it is more difficult to perform than the head tilt–chin lift.

Practice both the head tilt–chin lift and the jaw thrust with a CPR manikin. To obtain a course completion card, you will need to demonstrate that you can open the airway using the head tilt–chin lift and the jaw-thrust.

This chapter presents the steps of CPR for an infant or child. For the purposes of basic life support (BLS), the term *infant* refers to a child less than 1 year old; *child* refers to a child who is 1 to 8 years old. For children more than 8 years old, follow the steps of CPR for adults (Chapter 2).

The Steps of CPR for Infants and Children
1-Rescuer CPR

The lone rescuer performs CPR in the sequence depicted in the pediatric Chain of Survival:

■ Try to prevent arrest

■ **If the infant or child becomes unresponsive, provide CPR for 1 minute**

FIGURE 2. Opening the airway with the head tilt–chin lift. Gently lift the chin with one hand and push down on the forehead with the other hand. **A,** Infant. **B,** Child.

A

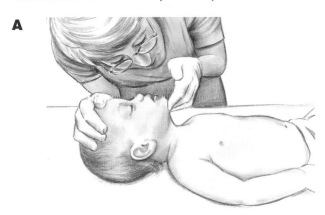

B

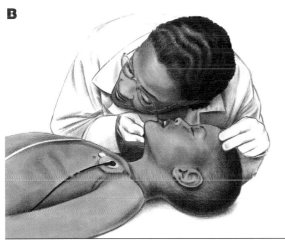

FIGURE 3. Opening the airway with the jaw thrust. Lift the angles of the jaw. This moves the jaw and tongue forward and opens the airway without bending the neck.

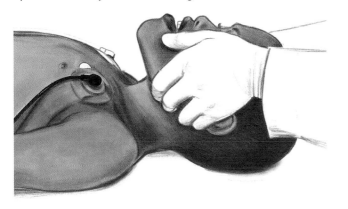

■ Phone the emergency response number. Remember: Begin the steps of CPR when you find an unresponsive infant or child.

1. **Check response: Check whether the victim is responsive by gently tapping the victim** and shouting "Are you OK?"

FIGURE 4. Obstruction of the airway relieved by positioning. **A,** In an unresponsive infant the prominent occiput flexes the neck, and the airway can become obstructed. Airway obstruction also can be caused by the tongue falling back against the throat. **B,** Position the infant with the neck in a neutral position so that the tragus of the ear is level with the top of the shoulder. This position will keep the airway open.

A

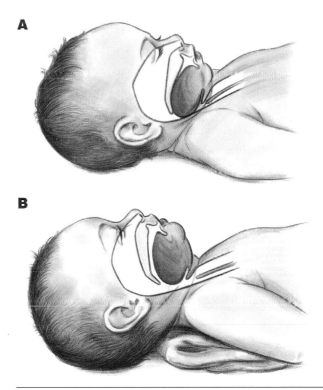

B

■ If the victim is *unresponsive*, **shout for help and begin CPR.** If anyone responds to your shout, tell that person to phone the emergency response number. This call activates the hospital response or emergency medical services (EMS) system and ensures that help is on the way.

■ **If you are alone** and find an unresponsive infant or child, **begin CPR.** Perform CPR for 1 minute. Then leave the victim and phone the emergency response number. An AED may be used for children 1 to 8 years of age after 1 minute of CPR.

■ Kneel at the victim's side near the head. The victim should be lying supine (on the back) on a firm surface (the floor is best). Carefully turn the victim onto the back if needed. Support the head and neck as you turn the victim. If you think the victim is injured, turn the head, neck, and back as a unit.

2. Airway: Open the airway.

■ *Head tilt–chin lift:* Gently lift the chin with one hand and push down on the forehead with your other hand (Figure 2). To lift the chin, place your fingers on the bony part of the chin. Avoid compressing the soft tissues of the neck or the area under the chin. Lifting the chin moves the tongue away from the back of the throat and opens the airway.

■ *Jaw thrust:* If you think the victim has a head or neck injury, use the jaw thrust to open the airway. Lift the angles of the jaw. Lifting the angles of the jaw moves the jaw and tongue forward and opens the airway without bending the neck (Figure 3).

3. Breathing: Hold the airway open and look, listen, and feel to determine if the victim is breathing adequately (Figure 2A and 2B). If the victim is not breathing adequately, give 2 rescue breaths.

To check for adequate breathing, *look, listen,* and *feel* for breathing:

a. Place your ear next to the victim's mouth and nose and turn your head to look at the chest.

b. **Look** for the chest to rise. **Listen** and **feel** for air movement on your cheek.

c. If the infant or child is gasping or breathing *very* slowly, breathing is inadequate. Treat the child as if he is not breathing at all.

If the victim is not breathing adequately, give 2 rescue breaths (Figure 5).

To perform rescue breathing in an infant (Figure 5):

a. Cover the infant's mouth and nose with your mouth (Figure 5). If your mouth is too small to cover the infant's nose and mouth, cover the infant's nose with your mouth and deliver breaths through the infant's nose. You may need to hold the infant's mouth closed to prevent air from escaping.

b. Continue to open the airway by tilting the head and lifting the chin (or perform the jaw thrust).

c. Give 2 slow breaths (1 to 1½ seconds each).

d. Be sure the infant's chest rises each time you give a rescue breath. The chest will rise if you are delivering enough air into the infant's lungs. Deliver just enough air to cause the infant's chest to rise. If the chest does not rise, reopen the airway and give rescue breaths again.

e. If a barrier device suitable for infants is available, use it to provide rescue breathing (see Barrier Devices later in this chapter).

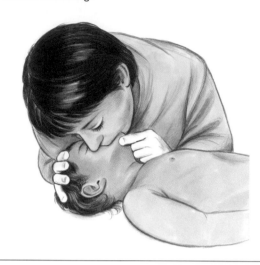

FIGURE 5. Mouth-to-nose-and-mouth rescue breathing for an infant. Place your mouth over the infant's nose and mouth. If you cannot cover both the nose and mouth, cover only the nose to provide rescue breathing.

To perform rescue breathing in a child (Figure 6):

a. Cover the child's mouth with your mouth and pinch the child's nose closed.

b. Continue to tilt the head and lift the chin (or perform the jaw thrust).

c. Give 2 slow breaths (1 to 1½ seconds each).

d. Be sure the child's chest rises each time you give a rescue breath. The chest will rise if you are delivering enough air into the child's lungs. If the chest does not rise, reopen the airway and give rescue breaths again.

e. If a barrier device suitable for children is available, use the barrier device to provide rescue breathing (see "Face Shields, Face Masks, and Bag-Mask Devices" later in this chapter).

4. Circulation

a. **Check for signs of circulation in response to the 2 rescue breaths.** Signs of circulation include pulse, adequate breathing, coughing, and movement. For an infant, check the brachial pulse in the arm (Figure 7). For a child, check for the carotid pulse in the neck (Figure 8).

b. Do not take more than 10 seconds to check for signs of circulation.

c. If you are not confident that signs of circulation are present, if you feel no pulse, or if you feel a pulse rate less than 60 beats per minute with signs of poor perfusion, begin chest compressions (Figure 9).

Foundation Facts:
Respiratory Arrest and Rescue Breathing

Respiratory arrest is present when the infant or child stops breathing or breathes so slowly, shallowly, or irregularly that delivery of oxygen to the heart and brain is severely reduced. *Remember. When breathing stops, delivery of oxygen to the heart and brain soon stops.* If oxygen delivery is not restored quickly, the heart and brain may be damaged. Rescue breathing is the fastest way to deliver oxygen to the victim's lungs and blood. Rescue breathing may prevent development of cardiac arrest.

You should have ready access to barrier and bag-mask devices to provide rescue breathing in the healthcare facility where you work. But at some time you may need to perform rescue breathing outside the hospital. For this reason you will learn to provide rescue breathing with the mouth-to-nose-and-mouth technique for infants and the mouth-to-mouth technique for children. You will also learn to use barrier and bag-mask devices to provide rescue breathing for infants and children.

When you provide rescue breathing, look to see if the victim's chest rises with each breath. Looking for the chest to rise is the only way you can tell if you are giving effective rescue breaths.

Deliver breaths slowly. Use just enough air to cause the victim's chest to rise. Take 1 to 1½ seconds to deliver each breath. Do *not* give rapid, large, forceful breaths. Forceful breaths will blow air into the stomach instead of the lungs. Air in the stomach (gastric inflation) can cause vomiting, which complicates CPR in many ways. *Remember: Your lungs hold much more air than an infant's or child's lungs. It is not necessary to blow a "full" breath for rescue breathing. Blow just until you make the chest rise.*

After you give 2 rescue breaths, check for signs of circulation. If you observe signs of circulation (pulse, adequate breathing, coughing, or movement in response to the rescue breaths), cardiac arrest is *not* present. But respiratory arrest may still be present. Be prepared to provide rescue breathing (1 breath every 3 seconds) if respiratory arrest is present.

When you *look, listen,* and *feel* for breathing and find that the victim *is* breathing adequately, do *not* give 2 rescue breaths. Watch the victim to be sure that breathing continues. If adequate breathing continues, place the victim in a recovery position to keep the airway open.

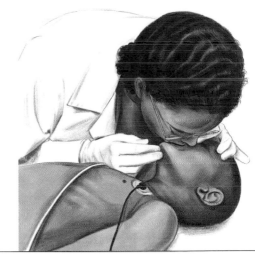

FIGURE 6. Mouth-to-mouth rescue breathing for a child. While keeping the child's airway open, cover the child's mouth with your mouth and pinch the child's nose closed.

FIGURE 7. Checking the brachial pulse in an infant. Feel for a pulse on the inner part of the upper arm between the elbow and the armpit.

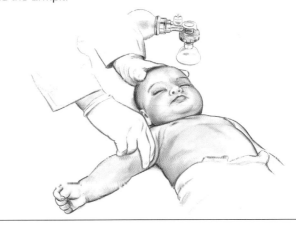

   d. Note: If the victim has signs of circulation (including a pulse rate greater than 60 beats per minute), chest compressions are *not* required. If the victim is not breathing adequately but signs of circulation *are* present, the victim is in respiratory arrest. Continue rescue breathing (give **1** breath every **3** seconds).

To provide chest compressions for an infant *if you are alone*, do the following:

   a. Imagine a line drawn between the infant's nipples.

   b. Place 2 or 3 fingers of one hand on the infant's breastbone (sternum) about 1 finger's width below the imaginary line (Figure 9). Continue to tilt the head with your other hand. Do not press on the very bottom of the breastbone (the xiphoid process).

FIGURE 8. Checking the carotid pulse in a child. **A,** Locate the Adam's apple with your index and middle fingers. **B,** Slide your fingers into the groove between the Adam's apple and the muscle at the side of the neck.

A

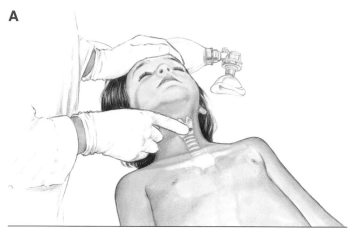

B

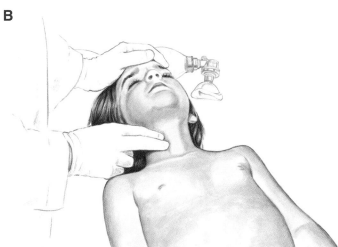

FIGURE 9. Two-finger chest compression technique for an infant. Note that the rescuer is using one hand to perform chest compressions and the other hand to hold the infant's head in a position that keeps the airway open. Holding the infant's head like this helps with delivery of rescue breaths.

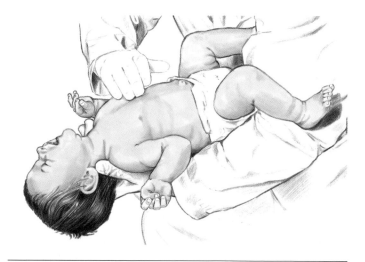

c. To provide compressions, press the infant's chest downward about *one third to one half* the depth of the chest. Provide compressions at a rate of at least 100 compressions per minute.

d. Release your pressure completely to allow the chest to expand after each compression, but do not move your fingers off the infant's chest.

e. Give **1** breath after every **5** compressions.

To provide chest compressions for a child (Figure 10), do the following:

a. Find the middle of the breastbone. Place the heel of one hand on the lower half of the breastbone (Figure 10). Do not place your hand over the very bottom of the sternum (the xiphoid process).

b. Continue to tilt the head with your other hand (tilting the head will keep the airway open and will help you deliver rescue breaths).

c. To provide compressions, press the child's chest downward about *one third to one half* the depth of the chest. Provide compressions at a rate of about 100 compressions per minute.

d. Release your pressure completely to allow the chest to expand after each compression, but do not move your hand off the child's chest.

e. Give **1** breath after every **5** compressions.

5. **Provide cycles of 5 chest compressions and 1 rescue breath.**

FIGURE 10. One-hand chest compression technique for a child. Note that the rescuer is using one hand to perform chest compressions and the other hand to hold the child's head in a position that keeps the airway open. Holding the head like this will help with delivery of rescue breaths.

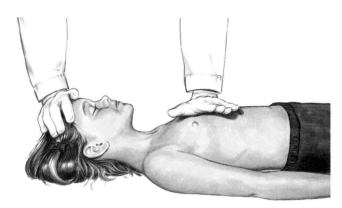

a. Continue to give 5 chest compressions and 1 slow breath.

b. After providing CPR for about 1 minute (about 20 rescue breaths or 20 cycles of 5 compressions and 1 breath; these will actually take a little longer than 1 minute), check for signs of circulation (adequate breathing, coughing, movement, and a pulse).

c. If no signs of circulation are present and no one has phoned for help, leave the victim and phone the emergency response number. If the child is small and uninjured, take the child with you. After you answer all of the dispatcher's questions, resume CPR.

d. An AED may be used for children 1 to 8 years of age with no response, no normal breathing, and no signs of circulation (including a pulse) after 1 minute of CPR.

e. Continue cycles of chest compressions and rescue breathing (5 compressions and 1 rescue breath) as needed. Check for signs of circulation every few minutes. If signs of circulation return, stop chest compressions and continue rescue breathing if needed (1 breath every 3 seconds).

2-Rescuer CPR

The skills used for 2-rescuer CPR for infants and children are essentially the same as those used for 1-rescuer CPR, but the skills are divided. When 2-rescuer CPR is performed, one rescuer kneels at the victim's head and the other rescuer kneels at the foot of the infant or the side of the child to perform compressions. The rescuer at the head performs all assessments and provides rescue breathing. The rescuer at the foot or side performs chest compressions.

The *2 thumb–encircling hands technique* (referred to as the 2-thumb technique) is the preferred compression technique for *infants* when 2 healthcare providers perform CPR (Figure 11).

Place both thumbs side by side or one on top of the other over the lower half of the infant's breastbone (sternum) about 1 finger's width below the nipple line. The nipple line is an imaginary line that connects the nipples. Be sure that your thumbs do not compress on or near the bottom of the sternum (xiphoid process). Encircle the infant's chest with the remaining fingers of both hands. Use both thumbs to compress the infant's sternum. Compress one third to one half the depth of the infant's chest. This depth corresponds to a depth of about ½ to 1 inch, but these measurements are not precise. After each compression completely release the pressure on the sternum and allow the sternum to return to its normal position. Do not lift your thumbs off the infant's chest. Deliver compressions for infants at a rate of at least 100 compressions per minute.

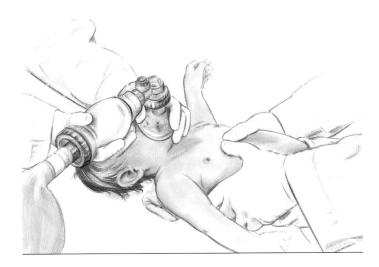

FIGURE 11. Two thumb–encircling hands technique. This compression technique is preferred for infants when 2 health-care providers are present.

To perform 2-rescuer CPR for a child, the rescuer performing chest compressions kneels at the side of the child's chest. That rescuer performs chest compressions using the same technique used for 1-rescuer CPR (the 1-handed technique). Deliver compressions at a rate of about 100 compressions per minute for children.

The compression-ventilation ratio (ratio of chest compressions to rescue breaths) is 5:1 for 1- or 2-rescuer CPR for infants and children. After 5 compressions the rescuer performing chest compressions pauses, and the rescuer at the head delivers 1 slow breath (1 to 1½ seconds). This pause is not necessary once the airway is intubated.

Continue providing CPR at a ratio of 5 compressions to 1 breath for approximately 1 minute (about 20 cycles of 5 compressions and 1 breath) as needed. Then have the rescuer at the head recheck for signs of circulation. If the child is 1 to 8 years of age and has no signs of circulation, an AED may be used.

If either rescuer becomes tired, switch roles. Switch quickly to minimize the interruption in CPR. The best time to switch is when it is time to recheck for signs of circulation. If signs of circulation are still absent, continue CPR at a ratio of 5 compressions to 1 breath until advanced care personnel arrive.

Recovery Position

If the victim resumes breathing adequately, rescue breathing is no longer needed. Place the victim in a recovery position (Figure 12). If the victim is injured, leave the victim on his or her back and hold the airway open. Use a jaw thrust to reopen the airway if needed.

FIGURE 12. Recovery position. There are several recovery positions. Place the victim in a position that supports the head and neck in a neutral position. Make sure there is no pressure on joints and bony prominences.

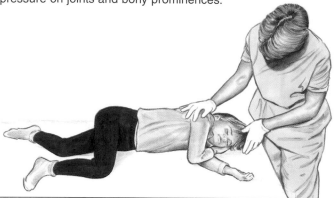

Face Shields, Face Masks, and Bag-Mask Devices

The American Heart Association recommends the use of barrier or bag-mask devices during rescue breathing. The Occupational Safety and Health Administration recommends that barrier devices (or bag-mask devices) be available in the healthcare facility and the workplace and that employees who perform CPR use these devices. A barrier device is not *required* to provide CPR. As of March 2000 there have been no reports of disease transmission during CPR training and no reports of spread of human immune deficiency virus (the virus that causes AIDS), hepatitis B virus, hepatitis C virus, or cytomegalovirus during performance of CPR.

Regardless of whether a barrier device is available, the key actions of the rescuer remain the same:

1. Open the airway using the head tilt–chin lift (or jaw thrust if the victim has a head or neck injury)

2. Provide rescue breaths (1 to 1½ seconds each).

When you use a barrier device, position the face shield or face mask over the victim's mouth and ensure an adequate air seal. *Deliver rescue breaths through the barrier device with just enough force to make the chest rise.*

There are 2 types of barrier devices, face shields (see Chapter 2, Figure 12) and face masks (Figure 13 in this chapter). Face shields are discussed in Chapter 2.

During this course you will learn how to use the barrier device that you will actually use in your workplace. Correct use of any barrier or bag-mask device requires practice. Practice on a manikin several times. The most critical step in using a face shield or mask is achieving a good seal around the mouth and nose. A good seal prevents leakage of air during rescue breaths.

FIGURE 13. Face mask. This barrier device is used to provide rescue breathing. Most face masks have a 1-way valve that prevents exchange of bacteria and viruses between the victim and rescuer. This valve must often be connected to the mask, so practice assembling the mask until you can do it in seconds. Most face masks can be connected to an oxygen source to enable mouth-to-mask rescue breathing with supplemental oxygen.

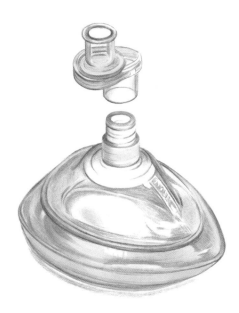

Using a Face Mask

Most face masks are stored in a plastic container or bag. Some masks require assembly before you can use them to provide rescue breathing. Become familiar with the face mask you expect to use *before* you need to use it. You must be able to assemble the device within seconds.

Rescuers who use a face mask kneel at the side of the victim (lateral technique) or at the top of the victim's head (cephalic technique).

Lateral Technique

The lateral technique is ideal for performing 1-rescuer CPR. To use the face mask, kneel beside the victim in a location that will allow you to perform both rescue breathing and chest compressions. Then do the following (Figure 14):

- Apply the mask to the victim's face. Use the bridge of the nose as a guide for correct positioning.

- Seal the mask. Place the index finger and thumb of the hand closer to the top of the victim's head along the edge of the mask. Place the thumb of your other hand (the hand closer to the victim's feet) along the lower edge of the mask.

FIGURE 14. Mouth-to-mask rescue breathing for a child, lateral technique. Press the mask firmly against the child's face while holding the airway open. Use the index finger and thumb of one hand to hold the mask against the bridge of the victim's nose. Also use this hand to tilt the head back. Use the thumb of the other hand to press the mask to the chin. Use the fingers of that same hand to lift the jaw up to the mask.

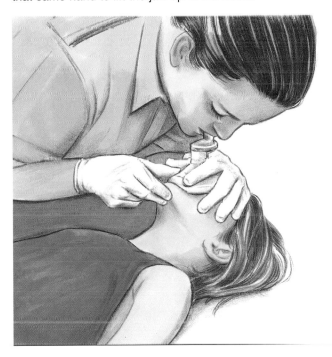

- Place the remaining fingers of the hand closer to the victim's feet along the bony part of the jaw and lift the jaw using a head tilt–chin lift.

- Compress the mask firmly around the edges to create a tight seal.

- Give slow rescue breaths. Be sure that the chest rises with each breath.

Cephalic Technique

Use the cephalic technique for 2-rescuer CPR or for 1-rescuer CPR when only rescue breathing is needed. There are 2 methods of holding the mask in place with the cephalic technique. Both methods are illustrated in Chapter 2 of this manual (see Chapter 2, Figure 14, B and C). To provide rescue breathing using the cephalic technique, kneel directly above the victim's head and do the following:

- Apply the mask to the victim's face. Use the bridge of the nose as a guide for correct positioning.

- Place your thumbs and the base of each thumb along the sides of the mask.

- Place both index fingers behind the angle of the jaw. Lift the jaw into the mask as you tilt the head back.

- While lifting the jaw, squeeze the mask against the victim's face with your thumbs and the heels of your hands. Squeeze firmly to achieve an airtight seal.

Provide slow rescue breaths (2 seconds each). Be sure the chest rises with each breath.

Bag-Mask Devices

Bag-mask devices consist of a self-inflating bag and a nonrebreathing valve attached to a face mask. (The nonrebreathing valve directs exhaled air from the victim into the environment so that the victim does not rebreathe exhaled air.) These devices are the most commonly used method of delivering rescue breathing both by EMS providers and in hospitals. Most bag-mask units have adequate volume to provide effective rescue breaths and make the chest rise.

Several studies have shown that rescuers in training often do not deliver adequate rescue breaths to manikins because they are unskilled in use of the device. A lone rescuer may have difficulty obtaining an airtight seal to the face while squeezing the bag and maintaining an open airway. If you are alone and you are having difficulty delivering rescue breaths that make the chest rise using a bag-mask device, check the following:

- Check the position of the head and neck. Reopen the airway.

- Check the seal between the victim's face and the mask. Be sure that you create a good seal between the mask and the victim's face. If a large amount of air is leaking, providing enough air to make the victim's chest rise will be difficult.

- Check the volume of the bag and the amount you are squeezing it. You may need to squeeze the bag more completely.

- Check the flow of oxygen into the bag. Make sure oxygen is flowing properly.

Because bag-mask ventilation is a difficult skill to master, bag-mask devices are most effective when 2 trained and experienced rescuers work together. One rescuer seals the mask to the victim's face and holds the airway open, and the other rescuer squeezes the bag slowly for 2 seconds (see below).

When you use a face mask or bag mask *with supplemental oxygen,* give slightly smaller rescue breaths (about 500 mL delivered over 1 to 2 seconds) than when you give rescue breaths *without* supplemental oxygen. You can give smaller breaths because the supplemental oxygen increases the amount of oxygen in the air the victim is receiving. Use of smaller rescue breaths reduces the chances of air entering the stomach, vomiting, and aspiration (breathing in of fluid or vomited material into the lungs). Smaller breaths are effective *only* if supplemental oxygen is used (minimum oxygen flow rate of 10 L/min for the face mask and 8 to 12 L/min for the bag mask). When you use a bag-mask device *with* oxygen, squeeze the bag slowly for 1 to 2 seconds until the chest rises.

Using a Bag-Mask Device

Rescue breathing with a bag-mask device requires instruction and practice. The rescuer must be able to use the device effectively in a variety of situations. Bag-mask devices come in many sizes, and you must select the appropriate size for the infant or child. Use of a device that is too large will increase the likelihood of air entering the stomach and aspiration.

If you are the only rescuer, kneel above the victim's **head** (Figure 15).

- If the victim has no head or neck injury, tilt the victim's head back. Place a towel or pillow under the head.

- Apply the mask to the victim's face with one hand. Use the bridge of the nose as a guide for correct positioning.

- Place the thumb and index finger of that hand around the top of the mask (forming a "C"), and use the third, fourth, and fifth fingers of that hand (creating an "E") to lift the jaw and hold the airway open.

- Maintain the head tilt and seal the mask firmly against the face.

- Compress the bag with your other hand. Watch the chest to be sure it rises.

- Deliver each breath for 1 to 1½ seconds. Maintain an airtight seal during delivery of each breath. If you do not have a tight seal, air will escape between the victim's face and the mask. Air leaks make delivery of effective breaths difficult.

Rescue breathing with the bag-mask device is most likely to be effective when 2 rescuers use the device as follows:

- One rescuer holds the mask against the victim's face and keeps the airway open. To hold the mask in place, use the techniques described for mouth-to-mask devices. To keep the airway open, use a head tilt–chin lift with a jaw thrust or use only a jaw thrust if a head or neck injury is present.

- The other rescuer squeezes the bag (Figure 16).

FIGURE 15. Use of a bag-mask device by 1 rescuer, E-C clamp technique. Using the thumb and index finger of one hand, form a C shape over the mask. Using the third, fourth, and fifth fingers, form an E along the jaw. Lift the jaw with the 3 fingers (the E) to keep the airway open (jaw thrust). Press down on the mask with your thumb and index finger (the C) to hold the mask in place. **A,** Infant. **B,** Child.

A

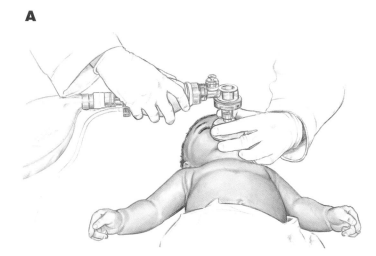

B

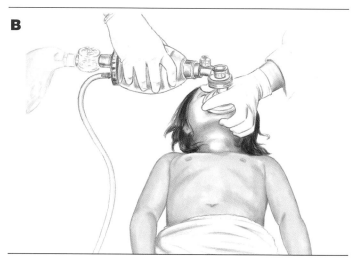

- If a third rescuer is present, that rescuer may apply cricoid pressure.

Bag-mask rescue breathing is a complex technique that requires considerable skill and practice. Practice using this device frequently.

Cricoid Pressure

Cricoid pressure prevents air from entering the victim's stomach. Use of this technique during rescue breathing reduces the risk of vomiting and aspiration. If a third rescuer is present, that rescuer applies pressure to the top of the victim's trachea (windpipe). This pressure pushes the trachea backward, compressing the esophagus against the

FIGURE 16. Use of a bag-mask device by 2 rescuers. One rescuer opens the airway (with a head tilt–chin lift plus a jaw thrust or a jaw thrust only) and holds the mask in place. This rescuer creates a tight seal between the mask and the victim's face and looks for the chest to rise. The second rescuer squeezes the bag. If a third rescuer is present and the victim is unresponsive, the third rescuer may apply cricoid pressure to compress the esophagus and prevent gastric inflation.

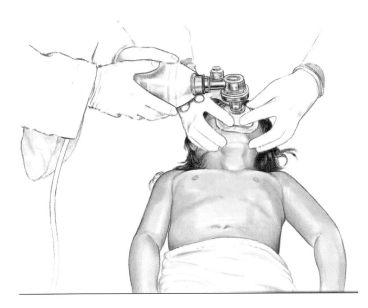

spinal column. When the esophagus is compressed, little air can enter the stomach. *Remember: Use cricoid pressure only if the victim is unconscious and only if 3 rescuers are present.* One rescuer performs rescue breathing, one performs chest compressions, and one applies cricoid pressure.

To apply cricoid pressure:

- Locate the thyroid cartilage (Adam's apple) with your index finger.

- Use your index finger to feel the "elevated area" below (cricoid cartilage).

- Using the tip of your index finger, apply firm backward pressure to this elevated area.

- Apply moderate rather than excessive pressure on the cricoid. Use of moderate pressure is particularly important if the victim is small.

Foreign-Body Airway Obstruction (Choking)

Foreign-body airway obstruction (FBAO) develops when an object becomes lodged in the airway and blocks the movement of air into and out of the lungs. If the blockage is severe or complete, the victim will be unable to breathe and oxygenate blood, and the brain, heart, and other vital organs will not have enough oxygen to function normally. If the blockage is not relieved, the victim will become unresponsive and can die.

Most episodes of choking in infants and children occur during eating or play, when parents or childcare providers are present. The choking event is usually witnessed, and the rescuer most often intervenes while the victim is still conscious and responsive.

Choking is an alarming and dramatic emergency. The desperate efforts of the choking infant or child to clear the airway heighten the emotional drama and increase the pressure on the rescuer to take the correct action.

How to Recognize Severe or Complete FBAO in a Responsive Infant or Child

Signs of severe or complete FBAO in infants and children include

- The *sudden* onset of respiratory distress associated with weak or silent coughing

- Inability to speak

- Stridor (a high-pitched, noisy sound or wheezing)

- Increasing respiratory difficulty

These signs and symptoms of airway obstruction may also be caused by infections such as epiglottitis and croup. Those infections cause swelling of the tissues in the airway so that the airway becomes very small. But signs of FBAO typically develop suddenly with no other signs of illness or infection, such as fever, rash, signs of congestion, hoarseness, drooling, lethargy, or limpness. Signs of *infectious* airway obstruction develop more gradually and are associated with other signs of infection.

The Heimlich maneuver (abdominal thrusts) and back blows and chest thrusts will *not* relieve infectious airway obstruction. A child with infectious airway obstruction requires immediate emergency care (phone the emergency response number or 911).

If an infant or child *suddenly* begins to cough, gag, or make high-pitched, noisy sounds, you should think that FBAO may be present. An older child may make the *universal choking sign* (hands clutching the neck) (Figure 17). Foreign bodies may *partially* block the airway but still allow adequate air movement. Victims with partial obstruction of the airway remain responsive, can cough forcefully (loudly), and usually can speak or cry. Breath sounds may be noisy, and you may hear wheezing between coughs. *If the airway is only partially obstructed, do **not** attempt to relieve the obstruction.* If you have any concern about the child's breathing, phone the emergency response number.

Victims with *severe or complete* FBAO will *not* be able to move enough air to make much sound. They will *not* be able to speak or cough forcefully. They may make very soft, high-pitched, or wheezing sounds when they try to inhale. When severe or complete FBAO is present you must act quickly to relieve the obstruction. Other signs of complete obstruction include signs that the infant or child is struggling to breathe (the ribs and chest sink in, or retract, when the infant or child tries to inhale) and blue lips and skin.

The following signs are *red flags* of severe or complete airway obstruction in a responsive infant or child. If you see any of the following signs, act immediately to relieve the obstruction:

- Universal sign of choking (hands clutching the neck [Figure 17]). Ask "Are you choking?" (The child may nod his head yes.) The infant will not make the universal sign of choking.

- Inability to speak, cough forcefully, or cry (the child may have ineffective, weak coughs). Ask "Can you speak?" (The child will shake his head no.) The infant will not make forceful sounds or cry forcefully.

- Weak, ineffective coughs.

- High-pitched sounds or no sounds while inhaling.

- Blue lips or skin.

FIGURE 17. Universal choking sign in a child.

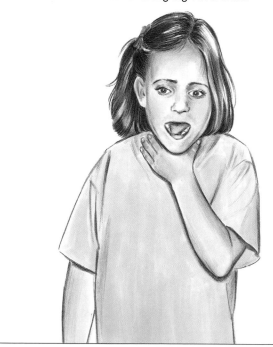

First Aid for Severe or Complete FBAO in the Responsive *Infant or Child*

This section first describes the actions you perform to dislodge a foreign body that is causing severe or complete airway obstruction in a *responsive* infant or child. Perform these actions when a responsive infant or child has signs of *severe or complete* airway obstruction and you think the obstruction is caused by a foreign body (for example, if a child who is playing with a small toy suddenly starts to cough forcefully and then cannot talk or make other sounds). If you do not act, the child may become unresponsive and may even die. **Do *not* follow these steps** if the cause of obstruction is *illness or infection* (for example, if the infant or child has been ill with asthma or has a "croupy" or hoarse cough).

Relief of Complete FBAO in a Responsive Infant

Do *not* give abdominal thrusts to an infant. Abdominal thrusts in an infant can damage the liver and other abdominal organs. To relieve FBAO in an infant, give 5 back blows and then 5 chest thrusts until the object is dislodged or the victim becomes unresponsive.

1. Hold the infant face down. Support the body with your forearm. The infant's legs will straddle your forearm. Hold the infant's jaw and support the head with your hand. Make sure the head is lower than the body. You may need to sit or kneel. Sitting or kneeling will allow you to rest the arm holding the infant on your lap or thigh.

2. Deliver up to **5** back blows with the heel of your free hand (Figure 18A). Strike the back forcefully between the shoulder blades. If the object is expelled and the infant begins to breathe with fewer than 5 back blows, discontinue the back blows.

3. If the obstruction is not expelled after 5 back blows, place your free hand along the infant's back and hold the back of the infant's head. The infant will be cradled or "sandwiched" between your 2 forearms.

4. Turn the infant's body as a unit so that the infant is lying on his back along your arm (the arm you used to give back blows). Support the head with the hand of the same arm. Keep the infant's head lower than the trunk.

5. Provide up to **5** quick downward chest thrusts in the same location as chest compressions — lower third of the breastbone (sternum), approximately 1 finger's width below the nipple line (Figure 18B). Chest thrusts are delivered at a rate of approximately 1 per second, each with the intention of creating enough of an "artificial cough" to dislodge the object.

FIGURE 18. Relief of severe or complete FBAO in a responsive infant. **A,** Back blows. **B,** Chest thrusts.

A

B

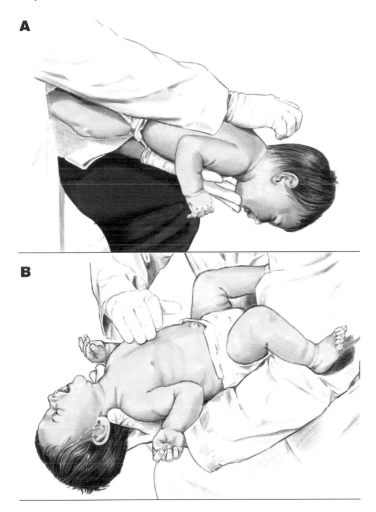

FIGURE 19. Abdominal thrusts (the Heimlich maneuver) in a responsive child.

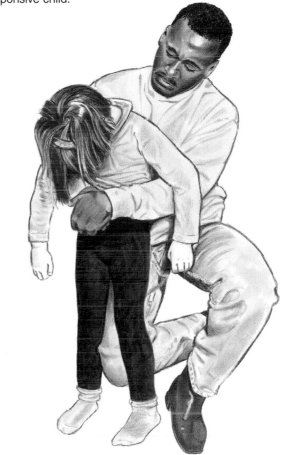

6. Alternate **5** back blows and **5** chest compressions until the object is expelled or the infant becomes unresponsive.

Relief of Complete FBAO in a Responsive Child

For children use the **Heimlich maneuver** (abdominal thrusts) to relieve complete FBAO. The Heimlich maneuver quickly forces air from the victim's lungs. The force of the Heimlich maneuver is similar to the force of a cough. The rapid air movement expels the blocking object like a cork from a bottle.

1. Once you determine that a child has severe or complete FBAO, tell the child you are going to help. Stand behind the child. Wrap your arms around the child (Figure 19).

2. Make a fist with one hand. Place the fist on the child's abdomen slightly above the navel and below the breastbone. Do not touch the bottom tip of the breastbone (the xiphoid process).

3. Grasp the fist with your other hand and deliver quick upward thrusts into the child's abdomen. Deliver several abdominal thrusts and watch to see if the object flies out.

4. Make each thrust a separate and forceful movement. Deliver abdominal thrusts until the object is expelled or the victim becomes unresponsive.

If complete FBAO is *not* relieved, the infant or child will become *unresponsive* and may turn blue. The infant or child may also stop breathing.

Sequence for Relief of FBAO in an Unresponsive *Infant or Child*

Victims of FBAO may initially be responsive when found by the rescuer and then become unresponsive. If this happens you will *know* the cause of the victim's symptoms. But if you find an unresponsive person you probably will *not know* that the victim has FBAO until repeated attempts at rescue breathing are unsuccessful.

Victims Who *Become* Unresponsive

Once the victim becomes unresponsive, he or she will not cough or attempt to expel the object. As soon as the victim collapses, look in the mouth and try to remove any object you see. To open the victim's mouth, use the *tongue-jaw lift*. Grasp both the tongue and lower jaw between the thumb and index finger and lift. This action moves the tongue away from the back of the throat (Figure 20). This action may partially relieve the obstruction. If you see a foreign body, carefully remove it.

Do not perform blind finger sweeps in infants and children. Blind finger sweeps may push the foreign body back into the airway and cause a worse obstruction. You may also injure the area above the glottis (the vocal apparatus of the larynx). If you open the mouth with a tongue-jaw lift and do not see any objects or if you removed an object and the victim is not breathing, give rescue breaths. If the rescue breaths are unsuccessful, reopen the airway and try to give breaths again. If rescue breaths are still unsuccessful, give alternating back blows and chest thrusts for infants or abdominal thrusts for children.

If you see the victim collapse and you *know* FBAO is the cause, follow this sequence of actions:

- Shout for help. If a second rescuer is available, send that rescuer to phone the emergency response number while you stay with the victim.

- Perform a tongue-jaw lift and look for the object in the back of the throat. If you see an object, perform a finger sweep to remove it. Do *not* perform a finger sweep if you do not see an object (Figure 20).

- Open the airway and give a rescue breath. If you are unable to make the victim's chest rise, reposition the head, reopen the airway, and give another rescue breath.

- If you still cannot deliver effective breaths (the chest does not rise), perform abdominal thrusts for the child and back blows and chest thrusts for the infant.

For the unresponsive child with FBAO:

- Straddle the victim's thighs (Figure 21) and give up to 5 abdominal thrusts (the Heimlich maneuver)

For the unresponsive infant with FBAO:

- Perform 5 back blows and 5 chest thrusts (Figure 18A and 18B)

Repeat the sequence of tongue-jaw lift, finger sweep (if object is visible), rescue breathing (attempt and re-attempt), and back blows and chest thrusts for the infant or abdominal thrusts for the child until the obstruction is

FIGURE 20. Tongue-jaw lift and finger sweep in an unresponsive victim of FBAO. To perform the tongue-jaw lift, grasp both the tongue and lower jaw between the thumb and index finger and lift to open the mouth. Look inside the victim's mouth for any visible objects. If you see an object, sweep the mouth with one finger to remove the object. Do not perform *blind* finger sweeps. That is, do not sweep the mouth without first looking inside it, and do not sweep the mouth if you do not see an object.

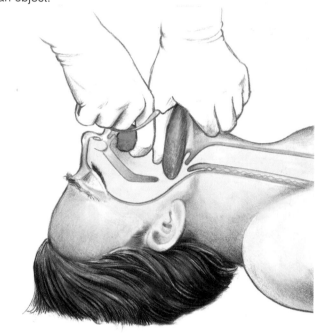

FIGURE 21. Abdominal thrusts in an unresponsive child.

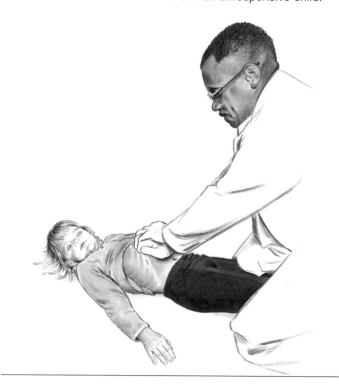

expelled and the victim resumes breathing or until the chest rises with rescue breaths. You may stop your efforts if advanced procedures are available to establish a clear airway.

Once the object is removed and the airway is cleared, check for breathing. If the victim is not breathing, provide slow rescue breaths. Then check for signs of circulation (pulse, adequate breathing, coughing, or movement). If there are no signs of circulation, begin chest compressions

If the chest rises during rescue breaths, check for signs of circulation. If the victim immediately begins breathing after the object is expelled, you may not need to check for breathing. If you are alone and the airway is not cleared after 1 minute, phone the emergency response number.

Victims Who Are *Found* Unresponsive

If you find an unresponsive person and *do not know the cause of unresponsiveness,* follow this sequence of actions:

- Shout for help. If a second rescuer is available, send that rescuer to phone the emergency response number while you stay with the victim.

- Open the airway and check for breathing (look, listen, and feel).

- If the victim is not breathing, attempt rescue breathing. If the victim's chest does not rise, reposition the head, reopen the airway, and attempt rescue breathing again.

- If you still cannot deliver effective breaths (the chest does not rise), perform abdominal thrusts for the child and back blows and chest thrusts for the infant.

- After each set of 5 back blows and 5 chest thrusts for the infant or 5 abdominal thrusts for the child, open the victim's airway with a tongue-jaw lift, look in the throat and remove any object you see.

Repeat the sequence of rescue breathing (attempts and reattempts), abdominal thrusts (back blows and chest thrusts for the infant), tongue-jaw lift, and finger sweep (if the object is visible) until the object is expelled and the victim resumes breathing, rescue breaths are effective, or advanced procedures are available to establish a clear airway.

Once the object is removed and the airway is cleared, check for breathing. If the victim is not breathing, provide 2 rescue breaths. Then check for signs of circulation (pulse, adequate breathing, coughing, or movement). If no signs of circulation are present, begin chest compressions. If the victim resumes breathing after the airway is cleared, you do not need to provide rescue breathing or check signs of circulation.

Presence of Victim's Family Members During Resuscitation

According to many surveys most family members would like to be present during the attempted resuscitation of a loved one. Parents and those who care for chronically ill children are often knowledgeable about and comfortable with medical equipment and emergency procedures. Family members with no medical background report that being at the side of a loved one and saying goodbye during the final moments of the victim's life is extremely comforting. Family members often fail to ask if they can be present during resuscitation attempts. We encourage you to offer this opportunity whenever possible.

Family members of victims who died after a resuscitation attempt report that being present during the resuscitation attempt helped them adjust to the death of their loved one. Psychological tests suggest that family members present during an unsuccessful resuscitation attempt have less anxiety and depression and more constructive grief behavior than family members not present during resuscitation.

When family members are present during resuscitative efforts, resuscitation team members should be sensitive to their presence. If possible one member of the team should stay with the family to answer questions, clarify information, and offer comfort.

Outside the hospital family members are typically present during resuscitation of a loved one. Outside the hospital healthcare providers are often too busy to attend to family members. But if you are able to provide brief explanations and the opportunity to stay with the loved one, you may be offering comfort to the family. Some EMS systems visit family members after a victim dies.

Stopping Resuscitative Efforts

Despite the best efforts of healthcare providers, most children who have a cardiac arrest do not survive. Return of spontaneous circulation is unlikely if the child does not respond to effective basic and advanced life support and 2 or more doses of epinephrine. Special resuscitation circumstances, local resources, and underlying conditions create a complex challenge for the resuscitation team. In the absence of a reversible cause of the arrest (such as a treatable arrhythmia, a history of a toxic drug exposure, or a primary hypothermic injury), the resuscitation team generally should discontinue resuscitative efforts after 30 minutes or less, especially if there is no return of spontaneous circulation. Chapter 8 discusses discontinuation of resuscitation and other ethical aspects of resuscitation.

Summary

This chapter described the assessments and skills of BLS for infants and children. There is no question that it is better to *prevent* a cardiac or respiratory arrest than to treat one. Healthcare providers must watch for signs of breathing difficulties or shock in infants and children. If you see a child in distress who may need advanced life support, notify your supervisor and activate the emergency response number. If respiratory or cardiac arrest does develop, be prepared to assess and support airway, breathing, and circulation. Your actions will "buy time" for the victim of cardiac arrest until advanced procedures can be provided.

Learning Checklist

Review the key information you learned in this chapter.

✔ The 3 red flags of cardiac arrest in an infant or child are

- No response to voice or touch

- No adequate breathing

- No signs of circulation

✔ When you encounter an infant or child in distress, perform the following actions first:

1. Determine responsiveness. If the victim is unresponsive, shout for help.

2. Open the airway and assess breathing.

3. If the victim is not breathing adequately, give 2 slow breaths. Make sure the chest rises.

4. Check for signs of circulation (adequate breathing, coughing, or movement in response to the 2 breaths or a pulse). If no signs of circulation are present or if you feel a pulse but it is less than 60 beats per minute in an infant or child with poor perfusion, begin chest compressions.

5. If you are alone with a child in respiratory or cardiac arrest, shout for help. If no one responds, give CPR for about 1 minute and then phone the emergency response number.

✔ Open the airway using the head tilt–chin lift. Use the jaw thrust if you think the victim's head or neck is injured. Then look, listen, and feel for breathing.

1. Turn your head to watch the chest: *Look for the chest to rise.*

2. Place your ear next to the victim's mouth and nose: *Listen for breathing.*

3. *Feel for air movement* on your cheek.

✔ If the victim is not breathing adequately, deliver 2 rescue breaths. Make sure the chest rises with each breath. After you deliver 2 rescue breaths, check for signs of circulation. If there are no signs of circulation (no breathing, coughing, movement, or pulse) or if you feel a pulse but it is less than 60 beats per minute in an infant or child with poor perfusion, begin chest compressions.

- In infants compress the breastbone (sternum) about 1 finger's width below the nipple line. In children compress the lower half of the breastbone.

- If 2 healthcare providers are present, use the 2 thumb–encircling hands technique for chest compressions in the infant.

- Do not press the very bottom of the sternum (the xiphoid process).

- In infants and children compress one third to one half the depth of the chest.

- Provide compressions at a rate of *at least* 100 compressions per minute for the infant and about 100 compressions per minute for the child.

- Provide 1 rescue breath after every 5 compressions.

✔ Use a compression-ventilation ratio (ratio of compressions to breaths) of 5:1 for infants and children.

✔ After giving CPR for about 1 minute, recheck the victim for signs of circulation and phone the emergency response number if that has not been done by another rescuer.

✔ The red flags of severe or complete FBAO are

- Universal choking sign (hands clutching the neck)

- Inability to speak, cough forcefully, or cry

- High-pitched or wheezing sound while inhaling

- Increased difficulty breathing

- Blue lips, tongue, and skin (cyanosis)

✔ To relieve complete FBAO in a responsive infant, give alternating sets of 5 back blows and 5 chest compressions until the object is expelled or the infant becomes unresponsive. If the infant becomes unresponsive, begin the sequence of actions for the unresponsive victim of FBAO.

✔ To relieve severe or complete FBAO in responsive children, give abdominal thrusts (the Heimlich maneuver). Stand behind the child. Make a fist and place it just above the navel and well below the breastbone. Place your other hand on top of your fist. Then deliver quick upward thrusts to the abdomen. Repeat abdominal thrusts until the object is expelled or the child becomes unresponsive.

✔ If the victim becomes unresponsive, begin the sequence of actions for relief of FBAO in the un-responsive infant or child. These actions include the tongue-jaw lift, looking for a foreign object, a finger sweep if an object is seen, back blows and chest thrusts for infants or abdominal thrusts for children, and rescue breathing (attempts and reattempts).

Review Questions

1. You are called urgently by a colleague working on the same floor. She is worried about her 2-year-old patient, who suddenly becomes limp. Which of the following steps do you take? Be sure to choose the correct order.

   a. verify that the child is unresponsive, phone 911 or other emergency number, check for signs of circulation, open the airway, give 2 breaths if needed

   b. open the airway, verify that the child is unresponsive, give 2 breaths if needed, check for signs of circulation, phone 911 or other emergency number if the child has no pulse

   c. verify that the child is unresponsive, tell your colleague to phone the emergency response number, open the airway, check for breathing, give 2 breaths if needed, and check for signs of circulation

   d. verify that the child is unresponsive, give 2 breaths, check for signs of circulation, phone 911, begin chest compressions

2. You are at the hospital cafeteria. A mother shouts that her child is choking and needs help. You run to the table and see an infant who is about 10 months old. The infant is awake and apparently struggling to breathe. She looks alarmed but is not making a sound. She is not coughing. Her lips are dusky. You see a plate with pieces of hot dog in front of the infant. The mother says the infant began coughing and gagging while eating the hot dog and then suddenly became silent. You tell the mother and the infant that you are going to try to help. What is your next action?

   a. give 5 back blows followed by 5 chest compressions until the hot dog is expelled or the infant becomes unresponsive

   b. give up to 5 abdominal thrusts (the Heimlich maneuver) until the hot dog is expelled or the infant becomes unresponsive

   c. attempt to provide rescue breathing

   d. open the airway and perform a blind finger sweep

3. You are unsuccessful in dislodging the hot dog, and the infant becomes unresponsive. You send the mother to phone the hospital emergency response number, and you lay the infant on the floor. You perform a tongue-jaw lift, and you see a piece of hot dog in the back of the infant's throat. You remove it, hold the airway open, and note that the infant is not breathing. What should you do next?

   a. give 2 rapid, forceful breaths

   b. give 1 slow breath

   c. check for signs of circulation

   d. give 2 slow breaths, making the chest rise

4. After you deliver rescue breaths, you check for signs of circulation. Which signs of circulation should you look for?

   a. the infant should have a pulse rate greater than 60 beats per minute and breathe adequately, cough, or move in response to the rescue breaths

   b. the infant should follow commands

   c. the infant should demonstrate the universal choking sign

   d. there are no reliable signs of circulation in the infant

5. You observe no signs of circulation, and you prepare to perform chest compressions. Which of the following responses gives the correct compression rate and compression-ventilation ratio for an infant?

   a. give 15 compressions and 2 ventilations at a compression rate of 60 compressions per minute

   b. give 5 compressions and 1 ventilation at a compression rate of no more than 60 compressions per minute

   c. give 15 compressions and 2 ventilations at a compression rate of 100 compressions per minute

   d. give 5 compressions and 1 ventilation at a compression rate of at least 100 compressions per minute

6. Where should you position your fingers to perform chest compression in this 10-month-old infant?

a. over a line drawn between the 2 nipples

b. 1 finger's width below the nipple line

c. 1 finger's width above the nipple line

d. over the very bottom of the breastbone (sternum)

7. What is the best sign that your rescue breaths are providing air to the victim's lungs?

a. the victim's color changes

b. the victim's pulse is visible on the neck

c. the victim's chest rises with each breath

d. you need medical equipment to determine whether you are providing air to the lungs

8. A child begins to cough forcefully and loudly while eating. What do you do?

a. give abdominal thrusts

b. give several back blows followed by several chest thrusts until the object is expelled or the child becomes unresponsive

c. phone 911 or other emergency response number

d. allow the child to cough and be prepared to act if signs of severe or complete FBAO develop

9. You are walking down the hallway of a hospital. You are called to the bathroom, where a 6-year-old with a known seizure disorder is reportedly unresponsive. Which of the following answers lists the most appropriate order of actions for you to take?

a. verify that the child is unresponsive and then ask someone to phone the emergency response number while you open the airway to assess breathing

b. begin rescue breathing, check for signs of circulation, determine the child's response to voice, and ask someone to phone the emergency response number

c. ask someone to phone 911 and position the child in the recovery position

d. perform abdominal thrusts (the Heimlich maneuver)

10. The 6-year-old child does not respond to voice or touch, takes only an occasional shallow breath, and has bluish lips. What do you do next?

a. begin chest compressions and ventilations at a ratio of 5:1

b. provide 2 rescue breaths and evaluate her response

c. position her in the recovery position and wait for EMS personnel to arrive

d. perform abdominal thrusts (the Heimlich maneuver)

How did you do?

1, c; **2,** a; **3,** d; **4,** a; **5,** d; **6,** b; **7,** c; **8,** d; **9,** a; **10,** b.

You are an emergency medical technician-basic (EMT-B) responding to a call about a nearby near-drowning. You arrive at the lake and find a young man swimming weakly and struggling to stay afloat in the water 50 yards from shore. You and your partner launch a dinghy into the water and quickly row out to the victim. Before you reach him the swimmer suddenly sinks below the surface. You manage to find him and pull him safely into the boat.

The victim is unresponsive. You open his airway and note that he is taking agonal breaths. You provide 2 slow breaths with a mouth-to-mask device and check for signs of circulation. He has no pulse or other signs of circulation. You start compressions while your partner dries the man's chest and attaches the AED. The AED indicates "no shock advised," but the victim still has no signs of circulation. You continue CPR while your partner rows the boat to shore.

Just as you arrive at the shore, the victim begins to move and cough and you note a carotid pulse. The young man becomes responsive during transport to the hospital. You think "Just in time! He's going to be all right."*

*From *BLS for Healthcare Providers,* Chapter 11: Special Resuscitation Situations.

Chapter 6

Special Resuscitation Situations

Overview

Several "special situations" can cause cardiac or respiratory arrest. These special situations require rescuers to change their approach to resuscitation. Such situations include hypothermia, submersion, trauma, electric shock, lightning strike, pregnancy, allergic reactions, and asphyxia. You must carefully note the differences in triage, emphasis, and resuscitation approach or priorities that are appropriate for these special situations.

Hypothermia

Severe hypothermia (body temperature below 30°C [86°F]) greatly reduces blood flow to the brain, heart, and other vital organs. It also greatly reduces blood pressure. The cold heart is extremely irritable and prone to development of deadly arrhythmias, particularly ventricular tachycardia and ventricular fibrillation (VF), if the patient is moved or stimulated excessively. The cold heart may not respond to defibrillation attempts until the core body temperature is above 30°C (86°F). When advanced cardiovascular life support (ACLS) is provided, the interval between doses of medication (for example, epinephrine) is increased to allow a longer time for the drug to circulate.

Victims can appear to be clinically dead because of marked depression of brain function and profound vasoconstriction. Successful resuscitation with full recovery is possible, but it is unusual. Full recovery has been reported among very small victims who cool quickly *before* the development of hypoxemia or cardiac arrest (for example, small children who are submerged in *icy* water or lost in the snow). In these victims the hypothermia reduces the oxygen requirements of tissues *before* hypoxia and respiratory and cardiac arrest develop. But victims of cardiac arrest may also develop hypothermia *after* the arrest. In these victims the hypothermia cannot have any protective effect. Instead it complicates management.

Learning Objectives

After reading this chapter you will be able to

1. Discuss the potential effects of severe hypothermia on the signs of circulation you are trying to assess

2. Describe BLS management of cardiac arrest associated with hypothermia

3. Explain the safety considerations associated with the rescue of a victim of submersion

4. Describe BLS management of cardiac arrest associated with submersion

5. Describe BLS management of cardiac arrest associated with trauma

6. Explain the safety considerations associated with the rescue of a victim of electric shock

7. Describe BLS management of cardiac arrest associated with electric shock or lightning strike

8. Describe BLS management of a cardiac arrest associated with pregnancy

9. Describe the special consideration for managing cardiac arrest associated with a severe allergic reaction

10. Describe the special consideration for managing cardiac arrest associated with asphyxia

The victim's pulse and respiratory efforts may be difficult to detect. Do not withhold lifesaving procedures because of this difficulty. Transport victims as soon as possible to a center where monitored rewarming can be performed.

Some clinicians believe that victims who appear dead after prolonged exposure to cold temperatures should not be considered dead unless they remain in cardiopulmonary arrest when they are warmed to near-normal core temperature. But when the victim of cardiac arrest is found in a cold environment (the arrest is unwitnessed), it may be difficult to determine if the arrest was caused by hypothermia or if the hypothermia followed the arrest.

Several years ago a very small toddler fell through the ice in a lake. The entire event was filmed by a news camera crew. When the child recovered some 30 minutes later, the child had normal neurologic function. The child was small and was cooled immediately by the submersion, and the cold water reduced oxygen demand. Contrast the hypothermia in the toddler with that in a middle-aged man who has a cardiac arrest while shoveling snow. The middle-aged man may cool down *after* the cardiac arrest. Hypothermia that occurs after cardiac arrest *complicates* the arrest and does not protect the brain during the arrest.

If you cannot determine which event occurred first (the arrest or the hypothermia), attempt CPR. If hypothermia is documented, take steps to limit heat loss and aid rewarming. Physicians in the hospital must use their clinical judgment to decide when resuscitative efforts should cease in a hypothermic victim of arrest.

Basic Life Support

The principles of care for the hypothermic victim who is *not* in cardiac arrest include the following:

- Prevent additional heat loss. Remove wet garments, cover the victim with layers of warm, dry blankets, and shield the victim from wind.

- Carefully transport the victim to the hospital. Avoid rough movement or activity that can trigger VF.

- Monitor core body temperature and cardiac rhythm.

- Do not delay urgent procedures, but perform them gently.

- Administer warmed, humidified oxygen. Additional warming techniques should be used only under controlled conditions in a medical facility.

When you find an unresponsive victim who may be hypothermic, begin the ABCs of CPR. Open the airway and look, listen, and feel for breathing. If the victim is not breathing, begin rescue breathing. Then check for signs of circulation. If the victim has no signs of circulation, provide chest compressions and prepare to use the AED. Remember to give 1 minute of CPR before using an AED for a child.

Allow yourself a longer time to check for signs of circulation (including pulse) and respirations because it is often difficult to detect shallow breathing or a weak pulse in a hypothermic victim with severe vasoconstriction. Take 30 to 45 seconds to detect signs of circulation (including a pulse and adequate breathing, coughing, or movement). If the victim has no signs of circulation, begin chest compressions.

AEDs should be available on virtually all BLS rescue units. AEDs may be used for victim 1 to 8 years old with no signs of circulation after 1 minute of CPR. Deliver up to 3 shocks in the hypothermic victim. If a shockable rhythm persists, stop defibrillation attempts and begin CPR, rewarming, and stabilization for transportation. If the victim's core temperature is below 30° C (86° F), successful conversion to normal sinus rhythm may not be possible until the victim is rewarmed. If the victim's core temperature is below 30°C (86°F), successful conversion to normal sinus rhythm may not be possible until the victim is rewarmed.

Critical Concepts:
BLS Care for Hypothermia

Following is a summary of general BLS principles for the management of victims of hypothermia:

- Remove all wet garments from the victim.

- Protect against heat loss and wind chill (use blankets and insulating equipment).

- Keep the victim in the horizontal position.

- Avoid rough movement and excessive activity.

- Administer warm, humidified oxygen (42°C to 46°C [108°F to 115°F]) if available.

- If the victim is not in cardiac arrest, provide passive rewarming if available.

- If cardiac arrest is present, provide chest compressions and ventilations, and provide up to 3 shocks with an AED. If the victim does not respond and the core body temperature is 30°C (86°F), continue CPR and stabilize the victim for transport.

Outside the hospital resuscitation may be withheld if the victim has obviously lethal injuries or if the body is frozen so completely that chest compression is impossible and the nose and mouth are blocked with ice. In the hospital physicians must use their clinical judgment to decide when to stop resuscitative efforts. Complete rewarming before pronouncement of death is not necessary for all victims. Predictors of outcome may be unreliable in the face of injury or other complicating factors. Because severe hypothermia is frequently preceded by other disorders (for example, drug overdose, alcohol use, or trauma), you must look for those underlying conditions and be prepared to treat them.

Submersion/Near-Drowning

For victims of submersion the length of time without oxygen is the main factor that determines survival. For this reason you must begin CPR as soon as possible. If you are alone, *perform CPR first* for about 1 minute before you phone 911 (or other emergency response number). Perform CPR first whether the victim is a child or an adult. CPR will deliver oxygen to the vital organs and may restore circulation and breathing. If a second rescuer is present, have that rescuer phone the emergency response number while you begin CPR.

Rescue From the Water

When you rescue a submersion victim from the water, you must ensure your safety first. Then ensure the safety of the victim. Get to the victim as quickly as possible. Try to bring some means of transport or a flotation device with you. Treat all submersion victims (particularly those who might have a diving injury) as though they have a head, neck, or spinal cord injury and avoid movement of the head and neck.

Rescue Breathing

Begin rescue breathing for the submersion victim as soon as you can safely reach the victim and open the victim's airway. In general use a jaw thrust to open the airway to avoid moving the head or neck. In this situation rescue breathing is most often started when the victim is pulled into shallow water or is pulled out of the water. If pinching the victim's nose, supporting the head, and opening the airway in the water are too difficult, you may perform mouth-to-nose ventilation as an alternative to mouth-to-mouth ventilation.

Injury to the spinal cord may occur when submersion followed diving or involved recreational equipment. You should also suspect spinal cord injury if the submersion episode was unwitnessed. If you think the victim has a neck injury or if the near-drowning episode was unwitnessed, keep the victim's neck in a neutral position (without flexion or extension). You can float the victim supine (face up) onto a horizontal backboard (support) before you remove him from the water. The rescue from the water should be done quickly so that you can begin CPR immediately. If the victim must be turned, align the head, neck, chest, and body; make sure the victim is well supported; and then "log-roll" the victim's head, neck, chest, and body as a unit. When you provide rescue breathing, be sure to keep the victim's head in a neutral position. Use the jaw thrust without head tilt or use the chin lift without head tilt.

Start rescue breathing immediately if the submersion victim is not breathing. Management of the airway and breathing for the submersion victim is similar to management of the airway and breathing for any victim in cardiac or respiratory arrest. Usual airway management devices, such as bag-mask ventilation, can be used. *You do not need to clear the airway of aspirated water* (that is, you do not need to perform the Heimlich maneuver) unless you cannot make the chest rise after multiple attempts to open the airway and provide rescue breathing.

Critical Concepts:
BLS Care for Submersion

Following is a summary of general BLS principles for the management of victims of submersion:

- When possible use a boat, raft, surfboard, or flotation device to rescue the victim from the water.

- Begin rescue breathing as soon as possible (in shallow water, in a boat, or on shore).

- If you suspect a spinal cord injury, keep the neck in a neutral position and quickly remove the victim using a spine board if available.

- Do not attempt chest compressions in the water. If compressions are needed, start them immediately after you remove the victim from the water.

- Do not attempt to drain water from the lungs.

- Remove foreign bodies (for example, seaweed, sand, or mud) from the airway.

- **Transport all submersion victims who require resuscitation to the hospital.**

Only a modest amount of water is aspirated by most drowning victims, and the majority of water is rapidly absorbed through the lungs. Use the Heimlich maneuver only if you think foreign matter is obstructing the airway and you are unable to make the chest rise with rescue breaths.

Chest Compressions and Defibrillation

Do not attempt chest compressions in the water. It is usually impossible to keep the victim's body horizontal and the head above water in position for CPR.

After you remove the victim from the water, immediately assess for signs of circulation. The pulse may be difficult to detect in a victim of submersion, especially if the victim is cold. If you cannot detect signs of circulation, start chest compressions at once.

Use an AED if there are no signs of circulation. AEDs may be used for children 1 to 8 years of age (about 9 to 25 kg or about 20 to 55 lb) after 1 minute of CPR. If the victim's core body temperature is less than 30°C (86°F), give a maximum of 3 shocks. If signs of circulation do not return after 3 shocks, resume BLS care until the core body temperature rises to 30°C (86°F) or more.

Transport all victims of submersion who require resuscitation to the hospital for evaluation and monitoring.

Cardiac Arrest Associated With Trauma

The rate of survival from out-of-hospital cardiac arrest caused by blunt trauma is uniformly low in children and adults. In some situations, both outside the hospital and in the Emergency Department, CPR is withheld when patients with *blunt* trauma are found in cardiac arrest. The rate of survival after cardiac arrest resulting from penetrating trauma is only slightly better. In victims of *penetrating* trauma (for example, gunshot or knife wound), rapid transport to a trauma center is associated with a better outcome than resuscitation attempts in the field. Some injured victims stop breathing but do not have a cardiac arrest. You will increase the victim's chance of survival if you begin CPR immediately. If you are alone and outside the hospital, *perform CPR first* for about 1 minute before you phone 911 (or other emergency response number) for a victim of trauma. Follow this sequence for victims of any age.

In injured victims damage to the jaw and facial bones may cause airway obstruction. If the victim sustains a head injury and becomes unresponsive, the tongue may block the airway. Immediately opening the airway and providing rescue breathing will increase the victim's chance of survival.

BLS for the trauma victim is otherwise fundamentally the same as BLS for a victim with primary cardiac or respiratory arrest. In victims of trauma rapid assessment and stabilization of airway, breathing, and circulation are the top priorities. You must also pay special attention to spinal immobilization (immobilize the head and neck), and you must stop severe external bleeding. Apply pressure to sites of bleeding.

Extrication and Initial Evaluation

When respiratory or cardiac arrest is present and resuscitation will be attempted, extricate the victim while protecting the cervical spine. Prepare the victim for rapid transport to a facility that provides definitive trauma care. Advanced care providers will assist in immobilizing the victim on a spine board, using lateral neck supports, strapping, and backboards throughout transport.

When there are multiple victims with serious injuries, emergency personnel must establish priorities for care. When the number of victims with critical injuries exceeds the capability of the EMS system, the victims without a pulse should be considered the lowest priority for care and triage. Most EMS systems have established guidelines that permit the out-of-hospital pronouncement of death or withholding of CPR when there are multiple victims with critical injuries or when victims have injuries incompatible with life. EMS personnel should work within such guidelines when available.

Establish Unresponsiveness

Head trauma or shock may cause loss of consciousness. If spinal cord injury is present, the victim may be conscious but unable to move. Monitor the victim's responsiveness. Check the airway, breathing, and circulation if the victim shows decreased responsiveness.

Airway

Immobilize the victim's spine throughout BLS maneuvers. Use a jaw thrust instead of a head tilt–chin lift to open the airway. If possible a second rescuer should be responsible for immobilizing the head and neck during BLS and until spinal immobilization equipment is applied.

Once the airway is open, clear the mouth of blood, vomitus, and other secretions. You can remove this material with a (gloved) finger sweep, or you can use gauze or a towel to wipe out the mouth. You may also clear this material with suction.

Breathing/Ventilation

If the victim is not breathing or has inadequate breathing (for example, agonal breathing or slow and extremely shallow breaths), provide rescue breathing. When you use a pocket mask or a bag-mask device, you must immobilize the cervical spine. Deliver breaths slowly to reduce the risks of gastric inflation (blowing air into the victim's stomach) and vomiting. If the chest does not rise despite attempts to open the airway and provide adequate ventilation, a tension pneumothorax or hemothorax may be present. These conditions require treatment by personnel with ACLS training.

Circulation

If the victim has no signs of circulation (no pulse and no adequate breathing, coughing, or movement in response to the rescue breaths), provide chest compressions and use an AED if available. AEDs may be used for victims 1 to 8 years old (about 9 to 25 kg or 20 to 55 lb) after 1 minute of CPR.

Apply pressure to stop external bleeding.

Disability

Throughout all interventions you must monitor the victim's responsiveness. Decreased responsiveness may indicate deterioration in respiratory, cardiovascular, or neurologic function. Be sure to reevaluate airway, breathing, and circulation.

Exposure

A victim of exposure may lose heat to the environment through evaporation. Such heat loss will be worsened if the victim's clothes are wet (for example, soaked with blood) or are removed. When possible keep the victim warm.

Electric Shock and Lightning Strike

Electric Shock

Most electric shock injuries in adults occur at work. Electric shock injuries in infants and children occur mostly in the home when the child bites electric wires, places an object in an electric socket, contacts an exposed low-voltage wire or appliance, or touches a high-voltage wire outdoors. Victims of electric shock can sustain a wide variety of injuries. Electric shock injuries range from an unpleasant tingling sensation caused by low-intensity current to cardiac arrest caused by exposure to high voltage or high current.

Lightning Strike

Lightning strike kills hundreds of people every year and injures many times that number. Thirty percent of lightning strike victims die, and up to 70% of survivors have lasting effects from their injuries.

The presentation of lightning strike injuries varies widely, even among groups of people struck at the same time. In some victims symptoms are mild and may not require hospitalization. Other victims die from the injury.

The primary cause of death in lightning strike victims is cardiac arrest. The cardiac arrest may be associated with primary VF or asystole. Lightning delivers an instant, massive countershock that disrupts the normal heart rhythm.

In many cases the heart rhythm may return spontaneously. But respiratory arrest caused by spasm of the chest muscles and suppression of the respiratory center in the brain may continue after the return of circulation. Unless rescue breathing is provided, the lack of oxygen may cause cardiac arrest.

The victims most likely to die of lightning injury if no treatment is given are those who suffer immediate cardiac arrest. Victims who do not suffer cardiac arrest and those who respond to immediate treatment have an excellent chance of recovery because delayed arrest is uncommon. When multiple victims are struck simultaneously by lightning, give highest priority to victims in respiratory or cardiac arrest. This triage priority is the opposite of triage priorities for trauma victims.

FIGURE 1. Pregnant victim placed in the left lateral position using overturned chairs for support. This position displaces the woman's uterus to the left side of her abdomen. To displace the uterus with the victim lying on her back, use gentle manual pressure.

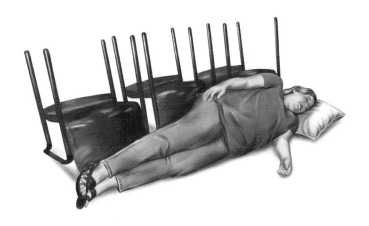

Modifications of BLS for Arrest Caused by Electric Shock or Lightning Strike

You must be certain that rescue efforts will not place you in danger of electric shock. Do not approach the victim of electric shock until *after* the power is turned off by authorized personnel or the energized source is safely cleared away from the victim.

Vigorous resuscitative measures are indicated even for victims who appear dead on initial evaluation. You should phone 911 (or other emergency response number), open the airway, assess breathing, and provide rescue breathing if needed. When electric shock occurs in a location not readily accessible, such as on a utility pole, start rescue breathing at once and lower the victim to the ground as quickly as possible.

If the victim has no signs of circulation (including no pulse), provide chest compressions and use an AED. AEDs may be used on victims 1 to 8 years old (about 9 to 25 kg or 20 to 55 lb) after 1 minute of CPR.

Be sure to protect and immobilize the spine during extrication and treatment if there is any likelihood of head or neck injury. Electrical injuries often cause related trauma such as injury to the spine and muscle strains and fractures because of the intense contraction of skeletal muscles. Remove smoldering clothes, shoes, and belts to prevent further thermal damage.

Pregnancy

CPR for pregnant victims is unique because of alterations in the mother's cardiovascular and respiratory physiology. During a normal pregnancy cardiac output and blood volume increase up to 50%. These changes make the pregnant woman more susceptible to and less tolerant of major cardiovascular and respiratory insults. Also, when the mother is supine the gravid uterus may compress the inferior vena cava and the abdominal aorta, decreasing blood return to the heart. This decrease in blood return can result in low blood pressure and even shock.

Causes of cardiac arrest during pregnancy include pulmonary embolism (a blood clot that travels to the lung), injury, severe bleeding related to delivery, amniotic fluid embolism (amniotic fluid that enters the bloodstream and travels to the lung), heart failure, abnormal heart rhythms, and heart attack.

To treat a distressed or compromised pregnant victim, place the victim in the left lateral position (Figure 1) or *manually and gently* displace the uterus to the left side of the abdomen. You can also use wedge-shaped cushions, multiple pillows, overturned chairs, a rescuer's thighs, or commercially available foam-cushion wedges (for example, the Cardiff wedge) to displace the uterus. Place the wedge under the victim's right abdominal flank and hip.

When cardiac arrest occurs in a pregnant woman, you should perform standard resuscitative procedures without modification except to displace the uterus to the left side of the abdomen. Use only the methods described to displace the uterus. Perform chest compressions slightly higher on the sternum because the uterus probably has pushed the diaphragm to a higher than normal position. Chest compressions will be most effective if performed with the victim propped on her left side with a hard surface behind her back.

Use an AED according to standard protocol. If the victim is outside the hospital and has refractory VF or other rhythms with a *"no shock indicated"* message on the AED, rapidly transport the victim to the hospital. In these victims emergency cesarean section may be performed to try to save a viable fetus.

Allergies

Severe allergic reactions are rare. But when they do occur the consequences may be life-threatening. Exposure to a known allergen (for example, foods or pollens) or a reaction to an insect bite (for example, bee stings) may be the cause. The most severe consequence of an allergic reaction is upper airway obstruction due to laryngeal edema or anaphylactic shock (life-threatening shock). If you think a person is having an allergic reaction, act promptly. Acting promptly can limit the adverse effects of an allergic reaction. After you phone the emergency response number, place the victim in a supine position and closely monitor the victim's airway. If respiratory or cardiac arrest occurs, begin rescue breathing or CPR. Some BLS healthcare providers can now assist patients in administering auto-injectable epinephrine for life-threatening allergic reactions.

Asphyxia

Asphyxia (suffocation) occurs when gas containing little or no oxygen is inhaled. Asphyxia may occur during fires, chemical spills, or gas leaks. It can also result from breathing carbon monoxide in an enclosed space. The result is insufficient oxygen to the body, which results in unconsciousness and ultimately cardiopulmonary arrest. The safety of rescuers at the scene is a priority. Ensure your own safety and then provide CPR. Always remove the victim from any environment with toxic gases. If the victim is breathing adequately or regains adequate breathing after resuscitative efforts, administer high-concentration oxygen as soon as possible. Victims of severe smoke inhalation may require transport to a tertiary care facility where therapies such as hyperbaric oxygen are available.

Exceptions to "Phone First" for Unresponsive Adults

If you are alone with an adult who is unresponsive, in general you should phone 911 (or other emergency response number) first and then begin CPR. In a small number of situations, you should first perform CPR (this may include rescue breathing alone or breathing plus compressions) for about 1 minute first and then phone 911. This approach will increase the likelihood of survival in victims with respiratory rather than cardiac arrest. Always direct a bystander to phone 911. But if you are alone, you should perform CPR for about 1 minute before you phone 911 if you think the unresponsiveness is caused by 1 of the following 3 conditions:

- Submersion

- Injury

- Drug overdose

Summary

Special resuscitation situations often require the rescuer to carefully assess conditions at the scene to ensure the safety of the victim and rescuers. Each special situation has important exceptions to the standard approach to a victim of cardiac arrest, but the basic actions remain essentially unchanged.

Learning Checklist

✔ In any special resuscitation situation you must assess the scene to ensure your own safety.

✔ Allow 30 to 45 seconds to assess breathing and signs of circulation in a victim with severe hypothermia.

✔ In victims of hypothermic cardiac arrest use of an AED outside the hospital is limited to 3 shocks to determine the victim's response to defibrillation. If 3 shocks do not result in effective defibrillation, continue CPR and transport the victim to the hospital.

✔ To prevent VF, avoid rough movement of and excess activity for hypothermic victims. Transport the victim in the horizontal position to avoid worsening hypotension.

✔ Always suspect spinal cord injury in victims of submersion, especially if submersion is associated with diving, involves recreational equipment, or is unwitnessed.

✔ Start rescue breathing immediately for a submersion victim who is not breathing.

✔ Do not routinely use the Heimlich maneuver for victims of near drowning. Use this maneuver only if you think a foreign body is obstructing the airway and you cannot make the chest rise with rescue breaths.

✔ The prognosis is poor for victims of cardiac arrest caused by blunt or penetrating trauma. But in victims in respiratory arrest immediate rescue breathing can be lifesaving.

✔ When the number of victims with critical traumatic injuries exceeds the capability of the EMS system, victims without a pulse should be considered the lowest priority for care and triage.

✔ When possible use an AED for all adult victims of cardiac arrest in special situations. AEDs may be used for victims 1 to 8 years old (about 9 to 25 kg or 20 to 55 lb) after 1 minute of CPR.

✔ For victims of electrocution or lightning strike, vigorous resuscitative efforts are indicated, especially for those who appear dead on initial evaluation. The victims most likely to die of lightning injury if no treatment is given are those who suffer immediate cardiac arrest. When multiple victims are struck simultaneously by lightning, give highest priority to patients in respiratory or cardiac arrest.

✔ To perform CPR for pregnant victims, wedge a pillow under the victim's right abdominal flank and hip or manually displace the uterus to the left side of the abdomen. These measures will keep the uterus from interfering with blood return to the heart and cardiac output during CPR.

✔ Exceptions to the "phone first" rule for unresponsive adults are (1) submersion, (2) trauma or injury, and (3) drug overdose. In unresponsive adults with any of these conditions, provide 1 minute of rescue support (rescue breathing or breathing with chest compressions) before you phone 911. If a second rescuer is present, send that rescuer to phone 911 while you provide rescue support.

✔ Suspect spinal cord injury for victims of submersion, trauma, electric shock, and lightning strike.

Review Questions

1. You find an unresponsive 27-year-old man in the woods during the winter. His skin is cold and frozen to touch. You open the airway and discover that he is not breathing. You deliver 2 rescue breaths and assess signs of circulation. How long should you take to check for signs of circulation (including the carotid pulse) before you start chest compressions?

   a. 5 to 10 seconds

   b. 10 to 15 seconds

   c. 30 to 45 seconds

   d. 1 to 2 minutes

2. You see a 12-year-old boy 100 feet from shore on a lake. He appears to be struggling to keep his head above water. As you watch, his head sinks below the surface of the water. You immediately send a bystander to phone 911. If all of the following options are available to you, which is the best action for you to take next?

   a. swim to the victim and pull him to shore

   b. use a boat to rescue the victim

   c. wait for EMS personnel to arrive

   d. attach an AED

3. You have just removed a 10-year-old girl from the bottom of a swimming pool, and she is unresponsive. You send a bystander to phone 911, and you open the child's airway. You note that she not breathing and that she has water in her mouth. Which of the following is the next action you should take?

   a. quickly sweep the water from her mouth and begin rescue breathing

   b. perform the Heimlich maneuver immediately

   c. turn her on her side, allow the water to drain for 1 minute, and then start rescue breathing

   d. attach an AED if one is available

4. You stop to help at the scene of a car crash. You find a 24-year-old man who was ejected from his car, and he is not breathing. What is the best method for opening the airway of this victim?

   a. head tilt–chin lift

   b. head tilt without jaw thrust

   c. chin lift only

   d. jaw thrust without head tilt

5. While visiting friends you discover that their 2-year-old son has bitten into the electric cord of a lamp. Sparks fly and the toddler is jerking violently. His mouth is still in contact with the wire. Which of the following should you do *first?*

   a. open the airway and evaluate breathing

   b. disconnect the plug from the outlet and send your friend to phone 911

   c. hold the child and place something in his mouth to prevent him from biting his tongue

   d. begin CPR and attach an AED

6. A pregnant woman collapses in the office building where you work. She is unresponsive. You open her airway and find that she is not breathing. You deliver 2 effective rescue breaths and assess signs of circulation. She has no pulse and no breathing, coughing, or movement in response to the rescue breaths. You start chest compressions and cycles of compressions and ventilations. After about 1 minute a member of the security staff arrives with an AED. The security guard notes that the victim is pregnant and wonders if it is appropriate to use the AED. Which of the following would be the best response?

   a. use the AED as you would for any victim of cardiac arrest

   b. do not use the AED because shocks will hurt the fetus

   c. use the AED but give only up to 3 shocks

   d. place the pads of the AED higher on the chest to avoid injuring the fetus

How did you do?

1, c; **2,** b; **3,** a; **4,** d; **5,** b; **6,** a.

You are at the health club, and you hear a commotion in the weight room. You quickly respond and find a 52-year-old man who has collapsed while exercising. You note that he is unresponsive and send a worker to phone 911. You open the man's airway and discover that he is not breathing. You have no barrier device. Will you perform mouth-to-mouth breathing on this stranger? If not, what are your options?*

*From *BLS for Healthcare Providers*, Chapter 10: Safety During CPR Training and Actual Rescue.

Safety During CPR Training and Actual Rescue

Overview

Questions about safety during CPR training and actual rescues are always asked during training courses. The general public may have concerns about the possibility of disease transmission or may be misinformed. This chapter clarifies the facts about disease transmission and describes the precautions you must take to reduce the very small risk of infection during CPR training and performance. Recommendations for manikin decontamination and rescuer safety were originally established in 1978 by the Centers for Disease Control and Prevention (CDC). Those recommendations have been updated twice by the American Heart Association (AHA), the American Red Cross, and the CDC. The current recommendations are discussed here and in the instructor's manual.

Disease Transmission During CPR Training

When you take a course in CPR, your risk of "catching" an infectious disease is extremely low. *Use of CPR manikins has never caused an outbreak of infection, and no cases of infection associated with CPR training have ever been reported. To date about 70 million Americans have had direct contact with manikins during CPR training with no reported cases of infection.*

Under certain circumstances infectious agents can live on manikin surfaces, presenting a possibility of disease transmission. Manikin surfaces should be cleaned and disinfected in a consistent way after each use by a rescuer and after each class.

Two important practices will minimize your risk of infection during CPR training. First, avoid contact with any saliva or body fluids present on the manikin. Your hands, lips, or mouth can become contaminated if you touch a manikin that has not been properly cleaned

Learning Objectives

After reading this chapter you will be able to

1. Discuss the risk of disease transmission during the performance of CPR

2. List methods for reducing the chance of disease transmission during the performance of CPR

3. Discuss the risk of disease transmission during CPR manikin practice

4. List methods for reducing the chance of disease transmission during CPR manikin practice

5. Discuss the benefits of face shields and face masks during the performance of CPR

between uses. This type of contamination can occur if you touch a manikin around the mouth before the manikin has been properly cleaned, if you practice mouth-to-mouth ventilation on a manikin that has not been properly cleaned, or if you place your fingers inside the mouth of the manikin during a practice session (for example, to demonstrate a finger sweep).

Most of this contamination will be prevented by adequate cleansing of the manikin between uses. But student rescuers often forget that when a manikin is used to practice mouth-to-mouth ventilation, the inside of the manikin mouth is contaminated with saliva unless it is cleaned or replaced after every use. If you touch the inside of the manikin mouth, wash your hands thoroughly before continuing practice. Otherwise bacteria can be transmitted from your hands to other students or to your own oral, nasal, or ocular (eye) mucosa.

Second, the internal parts of the manikin, such as the valve mechanisms and artificial lungs, must be thoroughly cleaned between uses. If these parts are not dismantled and cleaned or replaced after class, they may become sources of contamination for subsequent classes.

A wide variety of manikins are commercially available, and it is impossible to detail here the cleaning required for each model and type. Carefully follow the manufacturer's recommendations for manikin use and maintenance. Several intermediate-level disinfectants will kill organisms that may be present on manikins after use. Do *not* use solutions containing iodine, formaldehyde, or glutaraldehyde to clean manikins. Iodine may stain or damage plastic materials. Formaldehyde and glutaraldehyde leave undesirable residues and odors that may adversely affect students.

There is no evidence to date that human immunodeficiency virus (HIV), the virus that causes AIDS, can be transmitted by casual personal contact, by indirect contact with inanimate surfaces, or by an airborne route. HIV is extremely susceptible to disinfectant chemicals and is inactivated in less than 10 minutes at room temperature by a number of disinfectants, including disinfectants recommended for manikin cleaning. If you carefully follow the current recommendations of the AHA and the manufacturer's instructions for manikin cleaning and decontamination, you will minimize the risk of transmission of HIV, hepatitis B virus (HBV), and bacterial and fungal infections. Guidelines for cleaning are discussed in detail in the *Instructor's Manual for Basic Life Support*.

The risk of transmission of any infectious disease by manikin practice appears to be very, very low. Although millions of people worldwide have used training manikins in the past 30 years, *no documented cases of transmission of bacterial, fungal, or viral disease by a CPR training manikin* have been reported. In the absence of evidence of infectious disease transmission, the AHA vigorously emphasizes the lifesaving potential of CPR and continues to recommend broad-scale CPR training.

Disease Transmission During Actual Performance of CPR

Healthcare workers and public safety personnel must often perform ventilation on persons unfamiliar to them. During any given day or week a layperson is far *less* likely to perform CPR than a healthcare provider. If a layperson does perform CPR, it will most likely be in the home, where 70% to 80% of respiratory and cardiac arrests occur and where the rescuer knows the victim.

The actual risk of disease transmission during mouth-to-mouth ventilation is very, very low. Only 15 cases of CPR-related infection have been reported in scientific journals in the past 30 years. None of these cases involved transmission of HIV, HBV, hepatitis C virus, or cytomegalovirus. Despite the remote chance of disease transmission during performance of CPR, fear of contracting a disease is common.

Laypersons, physicians, nurses, and even BLS instructors may be reluctant to perform mouth-to-mouth ventilation. The most commonly stated reason for not performing mouth-to-mouth ventilation is fear of contracting AIDS. But once you perform CPR, your attitude is likely to change. Of bystanders who performed CPR in one study, 92% stated that they had no fear of infectious disease, and virtually all (99.5%) indicated that they would perform CPR again. Researchers have found little reluctance among lay rescuers to perform CPR on family members.

If you respond to an emergency for an unknown victim, follow your personal moral and ethical values and your knowledge of the risks of various rescue situations. Assume that any emergency situation involving exposure to certain body fluids has the *potential* for disease transmission for both you and the victim. If you are unwilling or unable to perform mouth-to-mouth breathing, give chest compressions alone. Although rescue breathing and chest compressions are best, chest compressions alone will increase the victim's chance of survival, particularly if the victim has gasping breaths or if the time to defibrillation is likely to be short.

The risk of disease transmission is greatest for persons who perform CPR frequently. Healthcare providers, both in hospital and out of hospital, are at particularly high risk. Out-of-hospital emergency healthcare providers include paramedics, emergency medical technicians, law enforcement personnel, firefighters, lifeguards, and others whose jobs require them to provide first-response medical care, including CPR. Out-of-hospital providers must take appropriate precautions to prevent exposure to blood or other body fluids. Such precautions will reduce the risk of contracting a disease from an infected person so that it is no higher than the risk for those providing emergency care in the hospital.

The probability that any rescuer (lay or professional) will become infected with HBV or HIV as a result of performing CPR is minimal. Although transmission of HBV and HIV between healthcare workers and patients has been documented, transmission in those cases was a result of blood exchange or penetration of the skin by blood-contaminated instruments. Transmission of HBV and HIV infection during mouth-to-mouth resuscitation has not been documented.

The emergence of multidrug-resistant tuberculosis and the risk of tuberculosis to emergency workers is a cause for concern. Rescuers with an impaired immune system may be particularly at risk for many infections, including tuberculosis. In most instances transmission of tuberculosis requires prolonged, close exposure such as occurs in households. But transmission to emergency workers can occur during resuscitative efforts by either the airborne route or direct contact. The magnitude of the risk is unknown, but it is probably low.

If a caregiver performs mouth-to-mouth resuscitation on a person suspected of having tuberculosis, the caregiver should be evaluated for tuberculosis. Standard approaches to treatment of tuberculosis, based on the results of baseline skin tests, should be used. Caregivers with negative results on baseline skin tests should be retested 12 weeks later. Preventive therapy should be considered for all persons with positive results on the baseline skin test and should be given to all converters.

Performance of mouth-to-mouth resuscitation or invasive procedures can result in the exchange of blood between the victim and rescuer. Exchange of blood is especially likely in cases of trauma or if the victim or rescuer has breaks in the skin on or around the lips or soft tissues of the mouth. A theoretical risk of HBV and HIV transmission during mouth-to-mouth resuscitation exists, but disease transmission has not been reported.

Barrier Devices:
Face Masks and Face Shields

To absolutely minimize the risk of disease transmission between you and the victim, follow the precautions and guidelines established by the CDC and the Occupational Safety and Health Administration (OSHA). Use barriers such as latex gloves and manual ventilation equipment with valves that divert the victim's expired air away from the rescuer (for example, a bag-mask system).

If you have an infection that may be transmitted by blood or saliva, do not perform mouth-to-mouth resuscitation if other effective methods of ventilation are immediately available.

If you are alone and are unwilling or unable to perform mouth-to-mouth ventilation, at least phone 911, open the airway, and perform chest compressions until a rescuer who is willing to provide ventilation arrives or skilled rescuers (for example, BLS ambulance providers or paramedics) with the necessary barrier devices arrive.

Several devices have been developed to minimize the rescuer's risk of exposure to pathogens. If a mouth-to-mask device is unavailable and mouth-to-mouth ventilation would place you at risk, use a barrier device such as a face shield or face mask. Face masks may be more effective barriers to oral bacteria than face shields. All face masks with 1-way valves prevent transmission of bacteria to the rescuer's side of the mask.

Because the efficacy of face shields has not been proven, those with a duty to respond should learn how to use masks with 1-way valves and other manual ventilation devices. Masks without 1-way valves and inline filters (including those with S-shaped devices) offer little protection, and routine use of such masks by rescuers with a duty to respond is not recommended.

Intubation with tracheal tubes and other airway adjuncts obviates the need for mouth-to-mouth resuscitation. Intubation also enables ventilation that equals or is more effective than the use of masks alone. The AHA encourages early intubation by skilled providers when both equipment and experienced professionals are available. Resuscitation equipment that is contaminated with blood or other body fluids should be discarded or thoroughly cleaned and disinfected after each use.

Summary

The risk of disease transmission during CPR training and performance is extremely low. But healthcare providers have a responsibility to follow the first principle of medical care during training and resuscitation: "Do no harm." The simple practice of infection control during CPR classes and the use of body-substance isolation during the performance of CPR will help prevent the transmission of disease and facilitate the well-being of both victims and rescuers.

Learning Checklist

Review the key information you learned in this chapter.

- The chance of disease transmission during CPR training and actual rescues is very low.

- Clean and disinfect manikins after each use. Follow the manufacturer's instructions and the recommendations of the AHA.

- Never place your fingers in the mouth of a manikin during practice sessions unless the mouth has been cleaned or replaced between uses.

↙ If you are unwilling or unable to perform mouth-to-mouth breathing on a victim of cardiac arrest, give chest compressions alone. Chest compressions may help save the victim's life.

↙ When possible use a barrier device with a 1-way valve to perform rescue breathing.

↙ In a study of rescuers who performed mouth-to-mouth resuscitation in actual cardiac arrests, 99.5% indicated that they would do it again if needed.

↙ Mouth-to-mask breathing is more effective than bag-mask breathing in delivering adequate tidal volumes.

Review Questions

1. A 43-year-old man has collapsed on a bus, and you perform mouth-to-mouth breathing and chest compressions. After the rescue a family member tells you that the victim is HIV positive. Which of the following responses best characterizes your chance of contracting AIDS from this contact?

   a. very high

   b. high

   c. moderate

   d. very low

2. You are a dispatcher and you receive a call from the scene of a cardiac arrest. You try to give instructions in CPR, but the caller refuses to perform mouth-to-mouth breathing because he is afraid of "catching" an infectious disease. What is the next best action you can take at this time?

   a. convince the caller to overcome his fear

   b. direct the caller to open the victim's airway and then perform chest compressions only

   c. tell the caller to search for someone who is willing to perform mouth-to-mouth breathing

   d. advise the caller that he has a legal responsibility to act

3. You are practicing CPR on a manikin with a friend. You note that she performs a finger sweep deep into the manikin's airway immediately after you have practiced mouth-to-mouth ventilation on the same manikin. What should you do?

   a. advise your friend to wash her hands before continuing practice

   b. don't worry; a finger sweep does not present a risk of disease transmission

   c. don't worry; a finger sweep is a routine activity during CPR training

   d. advise your friend to soak her hand in bleach for 10 minutes

4. You are an emergency medical technician, and you are responding to a cardiac arrest call. What is the best way to prevent infection during rescue breathing?

   a. perform chest compressions only

   b. use a barrier device or bag-mask device

   c. place a cloth between you and the victim

   d. use the mouth-to-nose breathing technique

How did you do?

1, d; **2,** b; **3,** a; **4,** b.

You are working in the ED and have been involved in the attempted resuscitation of 3 members of a single family whose car was struck by a drunk driver. Despite heroic efforts on the part of the prehospital and ED providers, all 3 victims — a father and his 2 children — died. The man's wife (the children's mother) arrives in the ED and is told of the deaths of her husband and children. You are with her as she says her goodbye to her family and then leaves. For days after the experience you have trouble sleeping, and you relive the attempts to save the lives of that family, wondering what you could have done better. What are some steps you can take to help you deal with this experience?*

*From *BLS for Healthcare Providers*, Chapter 12: CPR and Defibrillation: The Human Dimension.

The Human Dimension of CPR: Psychosocial and Legal Issues

Outcomes of Resuscitation Attempts: Definitions of "Success"

Since 1973 more than 40 million people have learned CPR. Many public health experts consider CPR training the most successful public health initiative of modern times. Millions of people have learned the skills needed to save the life of a fellow human being.

Unfortunately your best efforts will often be unsuccessful. CPR attempts at home or in public help restart the heart and restore breathing only about 50% of the time, even in communities with the highest survival rates. Research tells us that training healthcare providers and lay rescuers to perform CPR will dramatically increase the number of survivors of cardiac arrest. Higher survival rates have been documented in airports, casinos, and other settings where CPR was started immediately and defibrillation occurred within minutes of collapse. But in many locations ideal conditions are not present, and the success of resuscitation varies.

Even when hearts can be restarted, only about half of the victims of witnessed cardiac arrest caused by ventricular fibrillation who are admitted to the ED and the hospital survive and go home. This means that most of the time your CPR attempts will be unsuccessful. We think it is important to briefly discuss the emotional reactions you and other witnesses may experience after a resuscitation attempt, especially when your efforts appear to have "failed."

Healthcare providers are often called on to perform CPR in the workplace or the community. You can be confident that you are now better prepared to do the right thing if an emergency occurs at work, at home, or in the community. Of course these emergencies can have negative outcomes. You and the emergency personnel who arrive to take over care may not save the victim's life. But your

Learning Objectives

After reading this chapter you will be able to

1. Explain how often cardiopulmonary resuscitation (CPR) restores a normal heartbeat and breathing in victims of out-of-hospital cardiac arrest

2. Give 2 different definitions of "success" in resuscitation

3. State the importance of debriefing after a resuscitation attempt

4. Explain the role of a debriefing facilitator

5. Know how to contact an appropriate support person after a resuscitation attempt

success will not be measured by whether a victim of cardiac arrest lives or dies. Your success will be measured by the fact that you tried. Simply by taking action, making an effort, and just trying to help you will be judged a success.

Stress Reactions

A cardiac arrest is a dramatic and emotional event, especially if the victim is a loved one. The emergency may involve disagreeable physical conditions, such as bleeding, vomiting, or poor hygiene. Any emergency can be an emotional burden, especially if the rescuer knows the victim. The emergency can produce strong emotional reactions in bystanders, lay rescuers, and healthcare professionals. Failed attempts at resuscitation can be extremely stressful for rescuers. A resuscitation attempt will be even more stressful for you if you provide CPR for a family member, friend, or coworker. This stress can result in a variety of emotional reactions and physical symptoms that may last long after the original emergency. These reactions are common and normal.

It is common for a person to experience emotional aftershocks when he or she has experienced an unpleasant event. Usually such stress reactions occur immediately or within the first few hours after the event. Sometimes the emotional response occurs later.

Psychologists working with professional emergency personnel have learned that rescuers experience grief, anxiety, anger, and sometimes guilt. Typical physical reactions include difficulty sleeping, fatigue, irritability, changes in eating habits, and confusion. Many people say they are unable to stop thinking about the event.

Remember that these reactions are *common and normal.* They do not mean that you are "disturbed" or "weak." Strong reactions simply indicate that this particular event had a powerful impact on you. With the understanding and support of loved ones the stress reactions usually pass quickly.

Techniques to Prevent and Reduce Stress in Rescuers, Families, and Witnesses

Critical Incident Stress Debriefings

Psychologists have learned that the best way to reduce stress after rescue efforts is very simple: *Talk about it.* Sit down with other people who witnessed the event and talk it over. Healthcare personnel are encouraged to offer emotional support to coworkers, lay rescuers, and bystanders after both successful and unsuccessful resuscitation attempts. More formal discussions should include not only the lay rescuers but also the professional responders.

In these discussions you will be encouraged to describe what happened. Do not be afraid of "reliving" the event. Although such a fear is natural, talking about the event is a healthy way to deal with and overcome your fear. Describe the thoughts and feelings you experienced during the rescue effort. Describe how you feel now. Be patient with yourself and others. Understand that most reactions will diminish within a few days. Sharing your thoughts and feelings with your coworkers, fellow rescuers, EMS personnel, friends, or clergy can prevent or reduce stress reactions and help with your recovery.

In healthcare facilities and some other locations (for example, the homes of high-risk patients or worksites), administrators, team leaders, or EMS directors may establish plans for formal discussions or debriefings after resuscitation attempts. Such sessions are called *critical incident stress debriefings* (CISDs) or critical event debriefings.

Teams of specially trained persons are available to organize and conduct these CISDs. Such persons are usually associated with hospitals, EMS services, employee assistance programs, community mental health centers, or public school systems. Other sources of psychological and emotional support are clergy, police chaplains, fire service chaplains, or hospital and ED social workers.

Critical event debriefings are a confidential group process. The facilitator leads and encourages participants to express their thoughts and feelings about the event. You do not have to talk during the debriefing. But if you do, what you say may help and reassure others. Rescuers and witnesses of an event can discuss feelings they experienced during and after the resuscitation attempt. These feelings may include guilt, anxiety, or failure, especially if the outcome of the resuscitation attempt was negative. Ideally the rescuers who were most involved in the resuscitation should be present at the debriefing. In some public access defibrillation programs, EMS personnel visit lay rescuers who were involved in the resuscitative effort.

Psychological Barriers to Action

This course is preparing you to respond to future emergencies. Although you are preparing yourself by taking this course, there is a chance that you will never need to use your skills. Many healthcare providers have never been close to a victim of cardiac arrest and have seen CPR performed only on television or in the movies. Reality is quite different. During this course and while reading this manual, you may have had some troubling thoughts.

Here are some of the common concerns healthcare providers express about responding to sudden cardiac emergencies:

■ *Will I really have what it takes to respond to a true emergency?* Any emergency involving a loved one will produce severe emotional reactions. Parents, for example, sometimes feel paralyzed during the first few moments of an emergency involving their child.

■ *Will I be able to take action?* and *Will I remember the steps of CPR and defibrillation?* These are common concerns. One way to reduce these concerns is to practice the steps of CPR frequently so that you feel very comfortable performing the skills.

What about the unpleasant and disagreeable aspects of performing CPR? Would you be able to perform mouth-to-mouth rescue breathing on a stranger? What if the victim is bleeding around the face? What if a victim vomits during CPR? Would bleeding or vomiting pose a risk of disease for a rescuer without a CPR barrier device?

Often friends, relatives, or coworkers will be with you at the scene of an emergency. If you respond and take action, these people will often be willing to help. But they may look to you for instruction. It may be difficult to act decisively at such an unexpected and challenging time.

There are no easy solutions to help someone overcome these barriers. Think through how you would respond if confronted with an emergency. Mental practice, even without hands-on practice, is a good technique to improve future performance.

The American Heart Association (AHA) Emergency Cardiovascular Care Committee encourages you to attend routine skills review and practice sessions at least every 6 months. The required renewal interval for this course is *every 2 years*. Review and practice sessions and renewal courses will strengthen your skills, build your confidence, and increase the probability of a smooth and effective resuscitative effort. Most CPR programs for healthcare providers will provide review sessions to help you remain focused on the task at hand: performing the links in the Chain of Survival (phoning 911 or other emergency response number, providing CPR, and using an AED) to save a life.

Legal Aspects of CPR

The AHA has supported community CPR training for more than 3 decades. In that time lay rescuers and healthcare providers have helped save thousands of lives.

"Good Samaritan" Immunity for CPR Performed in the Community

A healthcare provider can perform CPR without fear of legal action when serving as a *Good Samaritan*. Chest compressions and rescue breathing require direct physical contact between rescuer and victim. These 2 people, rescuer and victim, may be strangers. Too often the victim of cardiac arrest dies. In the United States people may take legal action when they perceive damage or think that one person has harmed another even if the harm was unintentional. Despite this litigious environment, CPR remains widely used and remarkably free of legal issues and lawsuits. Although attorneys have included rescuers who performed CPR in lawsuits, no Good Samaritan has ever been found guilty of doing harm while performing CPR.

All 50 states have Good Samaritan laws that grant immunity to anyone who attempts CPR in an honest, "good faith" effort to save a life. In most states Good Samaritan immunity also specifically includes the use of an AED in the community. A rescuer is considered a Good Samaritan if

- The rescuer is genuinely trying to help
- The rescuer's actions are reasonable (you cannot engage in gross misconduct)
- The rescue effort is voluntary (the rescuer is not paid for the resuscitative effort)

Under most Good Samaritan laws rescuers are protected even if they have had no formal CPR training. There has never been a lawsuit in which a rescuer functioning as a Good Samaritan was found guilty of harming a victim of cardiac arrest.

Decisions About Resuscitation

CPR, like all medical interventions, has indications and contraindications to its use. Ethical values, including the potential benefit to the victim and the victim's requests regarding its use, must be considered. But CPR is unique because there is no time for deliberation. Unlike other medical therapies, CPR is instituted without an order from a physician. The standard of care remains that CPR should be started promptly unless specific contraindications exist.

The term *No CPR* means that in the event of a cardiac arrest, no cardiopulmonary resuscitative measures are to be taken. If a person with a No-CPR order has a cardiac arrest, no further treatment will be provided. In some communities the term *DNAR* (Do Not Attempt Resuscitation) is used to indicate that CPR should not be started.

The physician must obtain informed consent to issue a No-CPR order or must provide informed disclosure in cases where it can be demonstrated that CPR is of no physiological benefit. The order should be discussed with the patient's family as appropriate.

Determination of Death Outside the Hospital

For patients who suffer sudden cardiac arrest, prompt initiation of CPR remains the standard of care except when rigor mortis, lividity, tissue decomposition, or obviously fatal trauma is present. Those conditions are considered reliable indicators of death. The presence of a serious, chronic, debilitating disease or the terminal stage of a fatal illness may be used as criteria for not providing CPR. Resuscitation is rarely successful in patients whose cardiac arrest is associated with trauma except under specific clinical conditions.

Emergency personnel should not start CPR for victims with valid No-CPR orders outside the hospital. Pronouncement of death requires direct communication with physician medical control unless local protocol dictates otherwise.

Brain death cannot be determined by out-of-hospital personnel, and pupil status or other evidence of neurologic activity should not be used for the determination of death outside the hospital. Patients who are hypothermic should be aggressively resuscitated even when long transport times are involved.

Discontinuation of Resuscitation in Hospitals

Hospitals are required by the Joint Commission on the Accreditation of Health Care Organizations to have written policies for No-CPR orders. These policies need to be reviewed periodically to reflect developments in medical technology, changes in guidelines for CPR, and changes in the law.

Hospital policies should state that the attending physician is required to write No-CPR orders in the patient's chart. The rationale for the No-CPR order and other specific limits to care should be documented in the progress notes. No-CPR orders should be reviewed periodically, particularly if the patient's condition changes and especially before the patient undergoes anesthesia.

Hospitals are now required to have advisers, such as ethics committees, to help resolve ethical questions and issues. Ethics committees traditionally have been consultative and advisory and have been effective in organizing educational programs and developing hospital policies and guidelines for CPR.

CPR in Nursing Homes

Nursing homes should develop and implement guidelines for providing CPR to or withholding CPR from their residents. Care plans for residents should be individualized because CPR may not be indicated for all residents. Guidelines for withholding or initiating CPR should be developed and should be based on clinical criteria and patient preferences. All patients should be encouraged to state clearly whether they prefer resuscitation if the need arises.

Community Systems for Communicating No-CPR Orders

There is often confusion about whether a No-CPR order is transferable from the hospital to an out-of-hospital setting. Out-of-hospital settings include homes, nursing homes, and public places. Identifying victims who have a No-CPR order is difficult outside the hospital. The most common way to communicate a No-CPR order is to use a standard form that is available from health departments, EMS agencies, or physicians. Bracelets, identification cards, and central registries are also used. Healthcare providers and patients should be educated about appropriate documentation and the authenticity of various No-CPR orders in their local system.

Sometimes a family member will demand CPR despite the presence of a well-documented No-CPR order at the scene of an emergency. It may be appropriate in such cases to begin resuscitation and transport the victim to the hospital. Treatment can be discontinued when the conflicts are resolved and the authenticity and legitimacy of the No-CPR order are validated.

Sometimes there is confusion about the difference between No-CPR orders and living wills. No-CPR orders are physician orders directed to healthcare personnel specifically to withhold CPR. Living wills are legal documents stating a person's preference for medical care to be followed if the person loses decision-making capacity. Living wills require interpretation and must be incorporated into a medical care plan. Generally if a living will is presented to personnel who are providing resuscitation outside the hospital, emergency treatment should be started or continued and the victim transported to the hospital for interpretation of the will.

State laws, local ordinances, and EMS policies on the applicability of living wills in out-of-hospital settings should be reviewed. Advance directives that include written notations by the victim or verbal requests by family members about what the victim would want generally do not meet the procedural requirements for withholding emergency medical care.

Summary

Be proud of your initiative to take a course in CPR. Be proud of your new skills as a rescuer who can perform CPR to save a life.

Despite all the excitement about CPR and public access defibrillation, there are limitations to what you can do. Your efforts will not always succeed. What is important is taking action and trying to help another human being. Some people must overcome psychological barriers to action if asked to respond to a dramatic emergency such as cardiac arrest. Many of these barriers will be reduced during this course and with frequent practice of CPR skills. Feel free to express your concerns openly during the course and the small-group sessions.

Be aware of the mental and emotional challenge of rescue efforts. You will have support if you ever attempt resuscitation. You may not know for several days whether the victim lives or dies. If the person you tried to resuscitate does not live, take comfort in knowing that in taking action you did your best.

Learning Checklist

Review the key information you learned in this chapter.

- CPR attempts are often unsuccessful. Your efforts to save a life will not always succeed.

- The best way to reduce stress after a rescue attempt is to talk about it.

- Formal discussions or debriefings after resuscitations are called critical incident stress debriefings.

- Some people must overcome psychological barriers to action if asked to respond to a cardiac arrest.

- There has never been a lawsuit in which a rescuer was found guilty of doing harm in attempting CPR on a victim of cardiac arrest when the rescuer acted as a Good Samaritan.

- Your success will be measured by the fact that you tried.

Review Questions

1. A coworker who helped you perform CPR 2 days ago says she is experiencing fatigue, irritability, difficulty sleeping, guilt, loss of appetite, anxiety, and depression. What is the most likely cause of these symptoms?

   a. heart attack

   b. a virus that she caught while performing CPR

   c. stress response

   d. heart failure

2. Your friend who is experiencing the symptoms described in Question 1 asks what she should do to address this problem. You suggest that she attend a group meeting led by a physician, social worker, or other professional in which she can express her feelings. What is this type of meeting called?

   a. critical incident stress debriefing

   b. psychological analysis

   c. biofeedback

   d. psychological ventilation

3. An emergency physician approaches you after an unsuccessful resuscitation attempt. He asks you how he and his associates can help to reduce your stress after the event. What role might you suggest for the physician that would be helpful to you and other rescuers after a resuscitation attempt?

   a. facilitator of a debriefing process

   b. observer of a debriefing process

   c. passive participant

   d. no particular role

How did you do?

1, c; **2,** a; **3,** a.

Comparison Across Age Groups of Resuscitation Interventions

CPR/Rescue Breathing	Adult and Older Child	Child (≈1-8 y old)	Infant (<1 y old)	Newly Born
Establish unresponsiveness, activate EMS				
Open airway (Head tilt–chin lift or jaw thrust)	Head tilt–chin lift (If trauma is present, use jaw thrust)	Head tilt–chin lift (If trauma is present, use jaw thrust)	Head tilt–chin lift (If trauma is present, use jaw thrust)	Head tilt–chin lift (If trauma is present, use jaw thrust)
Check for breathing: (**Look, listen, feel**) If victim is breathing: place in recovery position If victim is not breathing: give 2 effective slow breaths				
Initial	2 effective breaths at 2 sec/breath (unless oxygen available)	2 effective breaths at 1 to 1½ sec/breath	2 effective breaths at 1 to 1½ sec/breath	2 effective breaths at ≈1 sec/breath
Subsequent	12 breaths/min (approximate)	20 breaths/min (approximate)	20 breaths/min (approximate)	30 to 60 breaths/min (approximate)
Foreign-body airway obstruction	Abdominal thrusts	Abdominal thrusts	Back blows and chest thrusts (no abdominal thrusts)	Back blows and chest thrusts (no abdominal thrusts)
Signs of circulation: Check for breathing, coughing, movement, or pulse If signs of circulation are present: provide airway and breathing support If signs of circulation are absent: begin chest compressions interposed with breaths	Pulse check (healthcare providers)* Carotid	(Healthcare providers)* Carotid	(Healthcare providers)* Brachial	(Healthcare providers)* Umbilical
Compression landmarks	Lower half of sternum	Lower half of sternum	Lower half of sternum (1 finger's width below intermammary line)	Lower half of sternum (1 finger's width below intermammary line)
Compression method	Heel of one hand, other hand on top	Heel of one hand	2 fingers or 2 thumb–encircling hands for 2-rescuer trained providers	2 fingers or 2 thumb–encircling hands for 2-rescuer trained providers
Compression depth	≈1½ to 2 in (4 to 5 cm)	≈⅓ to ½ the depth of the chest	≈⅓ to ½ the depth of the chest	≈⅓ the depth of the chest for newly born
Compression rate	≈100/min	≈100/min	≥100/min	≈120 events/min (90 compressions/ 30 breaths)
Compression-ventilation ratio	15:2 (1 or 2 rescuers, unprotected airway) 12 to 15 breaths/min asynchronous with compressions (2 rescuers, protected airway)	5:1 (1 or 2 rescuers)	5:1 (1 or 2 rescuers)	3:1 (1 or 2 rescuers)

*Pulse check is performed as one of the signs of circulation assessed by healthcare providers. Lay rescuers check for other signs of circulation (breathing, coughing, movement).

Skills Performance Sheets

The skills performance sheets serve two purposes. First and most important, the participant should use them to prepare and reinforce essential skills. Second, they are used to evaluate participant performance for satisfactory course completion.

Integrated Skills Evaluation Sheets are preferred for evaluation of healthcare providers. *Note that the healthcare provider should be able to demonstrate rescue breathing with mouth-to-mouth (or mouth-to–nose-and-mouth) ventilation, mouth-to–barrier device ventilation (with and without oxygen), and bag-mask ventilation.* Healthcare providers should use the ventilation devices used in their healthcare settings to increase their familiarity and facility with that device.

For AED skills performance sheets, ask 1 participant to act as timekeeper. This participant should time the collapse-to-shock interval (should be less than 3 minutes for healthcare providers) and the AED arrival–to-shock interval (should be less than 90 seconds). An interval of less than 90 seconds from arrival at the victim's side to delivery of a shock confirms that the rescuer is able to operate the AED efficiently.

The Integrated Skills Performance Sheets are designed to create a streamlined approach to evaluation. To demonstrate successful course completion, the healthcare provider must be able to perform 17 skills (including rescue breathing: mouth-to-mouth, mouth-to–barrier device, and bag-mask ventilation). Evaluation of each individual skill would require excessive time and thus detract from the practice of skills. For this reason integrated skills checklists

have been developed as evaluation tools for the healthcare provider. These checklists are used to document the following skills demonstrations:

1. Integrated adult 1- and 2-rescuer CPR

2. Integrated rescue breathing and relief of adult FBAO in the responsive and unresponsive victim

3. Integrated adult mouth-to-mask ventilation and CPR with use of an AED

4. Integrated child mouth-to-mask ventilation and CPR with use of an AED

5. Adult bag-mask ventilation (to be demonstrated during the integrated scenario)

6. Integrated relief of child FBAO in the responsive and unresponsive victim, CPR, and rescue breathing

7. Integrated relief of infant FBAO in the responsive and unresponsive victim, CPR, and rescue breathing

8. Child bag-mask ventilation (can be demonstrated during the integrated scenario)

9. Infant bag-mask ventilation (can be demonstrated during the integrated scenario)

The instructor should copy and distribute these simple skills performance sheets at each class for use during participant preparation and peer practice sessions. Participants will benefit from a review of important skills before the class to establish mental imagery and sequencing before skills practice. The checklists can also reinforce skills after the CPR course.

Appendix B
BLS Performance Criteria

Healthcare Provider Skills Performance Sheet
Adult 1-Rescuer CPR
Performance Criteria

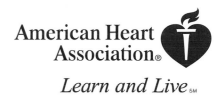

American Heart
Association®
Learn and Live ℠

Participant Name _____ Date _____

Performance Guidelines	Performed
1. Establish unresponsiveness. Activate the emergency response system.	
2. Open the airway (head tilt–chin lift or jaw thrust). Check breathing (look, listen, and feel).*	
3. If breathing is absent or inadequate, give 2 slow breaths (2 seconds per breath),† ensure adequate chest rise, and allow for exhalation between breaths.	
4. Check for carotid pulse and other signs of circulation (breathing, coughing, or movement in response to the 2 rescue breaths). If signs of circulation are present but breathing is absent or inadequate, provide rescue breathing (1 breath every 5 seconds, about 10 to 12 breaths per minute).†	
5. If no signs of circulation are present, begin cycles of 15 chest compressions (rate of about 100 compressions per minute) followed by 2 slow breaths.†	
6. After 4 cycles of compressions and ventilations (15:2 ratio, about 1 minute), recheck for carotid pulse and other signs of circulation. If no signs of circulation are present, continue 15:2 cycles of compressions and ventilations, beginning with chest compressions. If signs of circulation are present but breathing is absent or inadequate, continue rescue breathing (1 breath every 5 seconds, or about 10 to 12 breaths per minute).*†	

*If the victim is breathing or resumes adequate breathing and no trauma is suspected, place in the recovery position.

†If mouth-to-mask or bag-mask ventilation is provided **with supplementary oxygen,** smaller tidal volumes can be used but the chest should still rise. If ventilation is provided and there is a pulse, monitor oxygen saturation (if available).

Comments _____

_____

_____

_____

Instructor _____

Circle one: Complete   Needs more practice

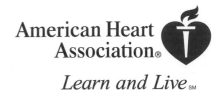

American Heart Association®

Learn and Live sm

Appendix B
BLS Performance Criteria

Healthcare Provider Skills Performance Sheet
Adult Bag-Mask Ventilation
Performance Criteria

Participant Name _____ Date _____

Performance Guidelines	Performed
1. Establish unresponsiveness. Activate the emergency response system.	
2. Open the airway (head tilt–chin lift or jaw thrust). Check breathing (look, listen, and feel).*	
3. If breathing is absent or inadequate, properly position the mask to achieve an effective seal while holding the airway open.	
4. Give 2 slow breaths (2 seconds per breath), ensure adequate chest rise, and allow for exhalation between breaths.*	
5. Check for carotid pulse and other signs of circulation (breathing, coughing, movement in response to the 2 rescue breaths). If signs of circulation are present but breathing is absent or inadequate, provide rescue breathing (1 breath every 5 seconds, about 10 to 12 breaths per minute).† If signs of circulation are absent, begin cycles of 15 chest compressions (rate of about 100 compressions per minute) with 2 rescue breaths.	

*If the victim is breathing or resumes adequate breathing and no trauma is suspected, place in the recovery position.

†If mouth-to-mask or bag-mask ventilation is provided **with supplementary oxygen,** smaller tidal volumes can be used but the chest should still rise. If ventilation is provided and a pulse is present, monitor oxygen saturation (if available).

Comments _____

_____

_____

Instructor _____

Circle one: Complete   Needs more practice

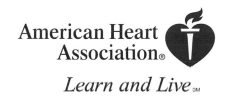

American Heart Association®

Learn and Live _{SM}

Appendix B
BLS Performance Criteria

Healthcare Provider Skills Performance Sheet
Adult 2-Rescuer CPR
Performance Criteria

Participant Name _____ Date _____

Performance Guidelines	Performed
1. Establish unresponsiveness. One rescuer should activate the emergency response system.	
Rescuer 1	
2. Open the airway (head tilt–chin lift or jaw thrust). Check breathing (look, listen, and feel).*	
3. If breathing is absent or inadequate, give 2 slow breaths (2 seconds per breath), ensure effective chest rise, and allow for exhalation between breaths.†	
4. Check for carotid pulse and other signs of circulation (breathing, coughing, or movement in response to the 2 rescue breaths). If signs of circulation are present but breathing is absent or inadequate, provide rescue breathing 1 breath every 5 seconds, about 10 to 12 breaths per minute).†	
Rescuer 2	
5. If no signs of circulation are present, give cycles of 15 chest compressions (rate of about 100 compressions per minute) followed by 2 slow breaths given by Rescuer 1.* Start compressions after chest rise (inspiration) from second breath.	
6. After 4 cycles of compressions and breaths (15:2 ratio, about 1 minute), Rescuer 1 delivers 2 rescue breaths and rechecks for signs of circulation (carotid pulse, normal breathing, cough, movement, or response to stimulation).* If no signs of circulation are present, continue 15:2 cycles of compressions and ventilations, beginning with chest compressions until an AED or emergency medical response team arrives.	

*If the victim is breathing or resumes adequate breathing and no trauma is suspected, place in the recovery position.

†If mouth-to-mask or bag-mask ventilation is provided **with supplementary oxygen,** smaller tidal volumes can be used but the chest should still rise. If ventilation is provided and a pulse is present, monitor oxygen saturation (if available).

Comments _____

_____

Instructor _____

Circle one:　　Complete　　Needs more practice

Appendix B
BLS Performance Criteria

American Heart Association
Learn and Live SM

Healthcare Provider Skills Performance Sheet
Adult FBAO in Responsive Victim
(and Responsive Victim Who Becomes Unresponsive)
Performance Criteria

Participant Name _____ Date _____

Performance Guidelines	Performed
1. Ask "Are you choking?" If yes, ask "Can you speak?" If no, tell the victim you are going to help.	
2. Give abdominal thrusts with proper hand position (chest thrusts for victim who is pregnant or obese), avoiding compressions on the lower sternum (xiphoid).	
3. Repeat thrusts until the object is expelled (obstruction relieved) or the victim becomes unresponsive.	
Adult Foreign-Body Airway Obstruction — Victim Becomes Unresponsive	
4. Activate the emergency response system.	
5. Open the airway with a tongue-jaw lift; perform a finger sweep to remove the foreign object.	
6. Open the airway and try to ventilate; if it is still obstructed (chest does not rise), reopen the airway (reposition head and chin) and try to ventilate again.	
7. If ventilation is unsuccessful, provide 5 abdominal thrusts with the victim supine. Ensure proper hand position, avoiding the lower sternum (xiphoid).	
8. Repeat steps 5 through 7 until rescue breathing is effective, then continue the steps of CPR as needed.*	

*If the victim is breathing or resumes adequate breathing and no trauma is suspected, place in the recovery position.

Comments _____

_____

_____

_____

Instructor _____

Circle one: Complete   Needs more practice

Appendix B
BLS Performance Criteria

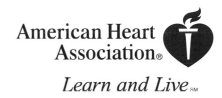
American Heart Association®

Learn and Live™

Healthcare Provider Skills Performance Sheet
Adult FBAO in Unresponsive Victim
Performance Criteria

Participant Name _____ Date _____

Performance Guidelines	Performed
1. Establish unresponsiveness. Activate the emergency response system. If a second rescuer is available, send that rescuer to activate the emergency response system while you remain with the victim.	
2. Open the airway (head tilt–chin lift or jaw thrust) and check breathing. If breathing is absent or inadequate, go to step 3.	
3. Attempt to ventilate; if unsuccessful (chest does not rise), reopen the airway (reposition head and chin) and try to ventilate again.	
4. If ventilation is unsuccessful, perform up to 5 abdominal thrusts with the victim supine. Ensure proper hand position, avoiding the lower sternum (xiphoid).	
5. Open the airway with a tongue-jaw lift followed by a finger sweep to attempt to remove the object.	
6. Repeat steps 3 through 5 until ventilation is effective (chest rises), then continue the steps of CPR as needed.*	

*If the victim is breathing or resumes adequate breathing and no trauma is suspected, place in the recovery position.

Comments _____

_____

_____

_____

Instructor _____

Circle one: Complete   Needs more practice

Appendix B
BLS Performance Criteria

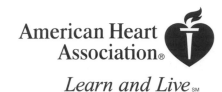

Healthcare Provider Skills Performance Sheet
Infant 1-Rescuer CPR
Performance Criteria

Participant Name _____ Date _____

Performance Guidelines	Performed
1. Establish unresponsiveness. If a bystander is available, send that person to activate the emergency response system.	
2. Open the airway (head tilt–chin lift or jaw thrust). Check breathing (look, listen, and feel).*	
3. If breathing is absent or inadequate, give 2 slow effective rescue breaths (1 to 1½ seconds per breath), ensure adequate chest rise, and allow for exhalation between breaths.	
4. Check for brachial pulse and other signs of circulation (breathing, coughing, or movement in response to the 2 initial rescue breaths). If signs of circulation are present but breathing is absent or inadequate, provide rescue breathing (1 breath every 3 seconds, about 20 breaths per minute).*	
5. If no signs of circulation are present or heart rate is less than 60 bpm with signs of poor perfusion, begin cycles of 5 chest compressions (2-finger technique, rate of at least 100 compressions per minute) followed by 1 slow breath.	
6. After about 1 minute of rescue support, check for signs of circulation.* If rescuer is alone, activate the emergency response system. If no signs of circulation are present (or heart rate is less than 60 bpm with poor perfusion), continue 5:1 cycles of compressions and ventilations. If signs of circulation are present but breathing is absent or inadequate, continue rescue breathing (1 breath every 3 seconds, about 20 breaths per minute).	

*If the victim is breathing or resumes adequate breathing and no trauma is suspected, place in the recovery position.

Comments _____

_____

_____

_____

Instructor _____

Circle one: Complete   Needs more practice

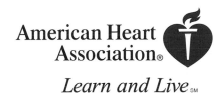

Appendix B
BLS Performance Criteria

Healthcare Provider Skills Performance Sheet
Infant Bag-Mask Ventilation
Performance Criteria

Participant Name _____ Date _____

Performance Guidelines	Performed
1. Establish unresponsiveness. If a bystander is available, send that person to activate the emergency response system.	
2. Open the airway (head tilt–chin lift or jaw thrust). Check breathing (look, listen, and feel).*	
3. If breathing is absent or inadequate, properly position the mask to achieve an effective seal while holding the airway open.	
4. Give 2 slow breaths (1 to 1½ seconds per breath), ensure adequate chest rise, and allow for exhalation between breaths.	
5. Check for brachial pulse and other signs of circulation. If signs of circulation are present but breathing is absent or inadequate, provide rescue breathing (1 breath every 3 seconds, about 20 breaths per minute).	
6. If signs of circulation are absent or heart rate is less than 60 bpm with signs of poor perfusion, provide 5:1 cycles of chest compressions and ventilations. If rescuer is alone, activate the emergency response system after approximately 1 minute.	

*If the victim is breathing or resumes adequate breathing and no trauma is suspected, place in the recovery position.

Comments _____

_____

_____

Instructor _____

Circle one: Complete   Needs more practice

Appendix B
BLS Performance Criteria

American Heart
Association®

Learn and Live ℠

Healthcare Provider Skills Performance Sheet
Infant FBAO in Responsive Victim
(and Responsive Victim Who Becomes Unresponsive)
Performance Criteria

Participant Name _____ Date _____

Performance Guidelines	Performed
1. Check for serious breathing difficulty, ineffective cough, *no* strong cry. Confirm signs of severe or complete airway obstruction.	
2. Give up to 5 back blows and 5 chest thrusts.	
3. Repeat step 2 until the object is expelled (obstruction relieved) or the victim becomes unresponsive.	

Infant Foreign-Body Airway Obstruction — Victim Becomes Unresponsive	
4. If a second rescuer is available, send that rescuer to activate the emergency response system while you remain with the victim.	
5. Open the airway with a tongue-jaw lift. If you see the object, remove it *(no blind finger sweeps).*	
6. Open the airway and try to ventilate; if still obstructed (chest does not rise), reopen the airway (reposition head and chin) and try to ventilate again.	
7. If ventilation is unsuccessful, give 5 back blows and 5 chest thrusts.	
8. Repeat steps 5 through 7 until ventilation is effective, then continue the steps of CPR as needed.*	
9. If the rescuer is alone and the airway obstruction is not relieved after about 1 minute, activate the emergency response system.	

*If the victim is breathing or resumes normal breathing and no trauma is suspected, place in the recovery position.

Comments _____

_____

_____

Instructor _____

Circle one: Complete   Needs more practice

Appendix B
BLS Performance Criteria

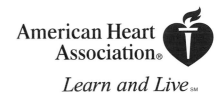
American Heart Association®
Learn and Live sm

Healthcare Provider Skills Performance Sheet
Infant FBAO in Unresponsive Victim
Performance Criteria

Participant Name _____ Date _____

Performance Guidelines	Performed
1. Establish unresponsiveness. If a second rescuer is available, send that rescuer to activate the emergency response system while you remain with the victim.	
2. Open the airway, check for breathing. If breathing is absent or inadequate, go to step 3.	
3. Attempt to ventilate if unsuccessful (chest does not rise), reopen the airway (reposition head and chin), and try to ventilate again.	
4. If ventilation is unsuccessful, give up to 5 back blows with heel of hand and 5 chest thrusts (use 2-finger technique).	
5. Open the airway with a tongue-jaw lift. If you see the object, remove it *(no blind finger sweeps)*.	
6. Repeat steps 3 through 5 until ventilation is effective, then continue the steps of CPR as needed.*	
7. If the rescuer is alone and airway obstruction is not relieved after about 1 minute, activate the emergency response system.	

*If the victim is breathing or resumes normal breathing and no trauma is suspected, place in the recovery position.

Comments _____

_____

_____

_____

_____

Instructor _____

Circle one: Complete   Needs more practice

Appendix B
BLS Performance Criteria

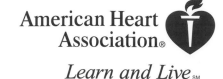

Healthcare Provider Skills Performance Sheet
Infant and Child 2-Rescuer CPR
Performance Criteria

Participant Name _____ Date _____

Performance Guidelines	Performed
1. Establish unresponsiveness. One rescuer activates the emergency response system.	
Rescuer 1	
2. Open the airway (head tilt–chin lift or jaw thrust). Check breathing (look, listen, and feel).*	
3. If breathing is absent or inadequate, give 2 slow breaths (1 to 1½ seconds per breath), ensure adequate chest rise, and allow for exhalation between breaths.	
4. Check for pulse (brachial in infants, carotid in children) and other signs of circulation (breathing, coughing, or movement in response to 2 rescue breaths). If signs of circulation are present but breathing is absent or inadequate, provide rescue breathing (1 breath every 3 seconds, about 20 breaths per minute).	
Rescuer 2	
5. If no signs of circulation are present, or heart rate is less than 60 bpm with signs of poor perfusion, begin cycles of 5 chest compressions and 1 breath. Pause to allow Rescuer 1 to provide 1 slow breath after 5 compressions.* Start compression at end of chest rise from rescue breath. • *Infants: use 2 thumb–encircling hands compression technique, compression rate of at least 100 per minute.* • *Child: typically use 1-hand compression technique, compression rate of about 100 compressions per minute.*	
6. After 20 cycles of 5:1 (about 1 minute), Rescuer 1 provides 1 breath and rechecks for signs of circulation (pulse, breathing, cough, movement, response to stimulation).* If no signs of circulation are present, continue cycles of compressions and ventilations (5:1 ratio), beginning with chest compressions.	

*If the victim is breathing or resumes normal breathing and no trauma is suspected, place in the recovery position.

Comments _____

Instructor _____

Circle one: Complete   Needs more practice

Appendix B
BLS Performance Criteria

Healthcare Provider Skills Performance Sheet
Child 1-Rescuer CPR
Performance Criteria

American Heart
Association®

Learn and Live sm

Participant Name _____ Date _____

Performance Guidelines	Performed
1. Establish unresponsiveness. If a bystander is available, send that person to activate the emergency response system.	
2. Open the airway (head tilt–chin lift or jaw thrust). Check for normal breathing (look, listen, and feel).*	
3. If breathing is absent or inadequate, give 2 slow effective rescue breaths (1 to 1½ seconds per breath), ensure adequate chest rise, and allow for exhalation between breaths.	
4. Check for carotid pulse and other signs of circulation (breathing, coughing, or movement in response to initial 2 rescue breaths). If signs of circulation are present but breathing is absent or inadequate, provide rescue breathing (1 breath every 3 seconds, about 20 breaths per minute).*	
5. If no signs of circulation are present or heart rate is less than 60 bpm with signs of poor perfusion, begin cycles of 5 chest compressions (typically 1-hand compression technique, rate of about 100 compressions per minute) and 1 slow breath.	
6. After about 1 minute of rescue support, check for signs of circulation.* If rescuer is alone, activate the emergency response system. If no signs of circulation are present, continue 5:1 cycles of compressions and ventilations. If signs of circulation are present but breathing is absent or inadequate, continue rescue breathing (1 breath every 3 seconds, about 20 breaths per minute).	

*If the victim is breathing or resumes normal breathing and no trauma is suspected, place in the recovery position.

Comments _____

_____

_____

_____

Instructor _____

Circle one: Complete   Needs more practice

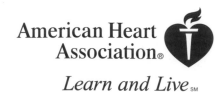

American Heart
Association®

Learn and Live sm

Appendix B
BLS Performance Criteria

Healthcare Provider Skills Performance Sheet
Child Bag-Mask Ventilation
Performance Criteria

Participant Name _____ Date _____

Performance Guidelines	Performed
1. Establish unresponsiveness. If a second rescuer is available, send that person to activate the emergency response system.	
2. Open the airway (head tilt–chin lift or jaw thrust). Check breathing (look, listen, and feel).*	
3. If breathing is absent or inadequate, properly position mask to achieve an effective seal while holding the airway open.	
4. Give 2 slow effective breaths (1 to 1½ seconds per breath), ensure adequate chest rise, and allow for exhalation between breaths.	
5. Check for carotid pulse and other signs of circulation (breathing, coughing, or movement in response to 2 breaths). If signs of circulation are present but breathing is absent or inadequate, provide rescue breathing (1 breath every 3 seconds, about 20 breaths per minute).	
6. If signs of circulation are absent or heart rate is less than 60 bpm with signs of poor perfusion, begin 5:1 cycles of compressions and ventilations. If the rescuer is alone, activate the emergency response system after approximately 1 minute.	

*If the victim is breathing or resumes normal breathing and no trauma is suspected, place in the recovery position.

Comments _____

_____

_____

_____

_____

Instructor _____

Circle one: Complete   Needs more practice

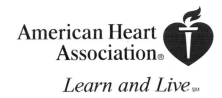

American Heart Association®

Learn and Live ℠

Appendix B
BLS Performance Criteria

Healthcare Provider Skills Performance Sheet
Child FBAO in Responsive Victim
(and Responsive Victim Who Becomes Unresponsive)
Performance Criteria

Participant Name _____   Date _____

Performance Guidelines	Performed
1. Ask "Are you choking?" If yes, ask "Can you speak?" If no, tell child you are going to help.	
2. Give abdominal thrusts using proper hand position (avoid xiphoid).	
3. Repeat thrusts until object is expelled (obstruction removed) or victim becomes unresponsive.	

Child Foreign-Body Airway Obstruction — Victim Becomes Unresponsive	
4. If a second rescuer is available, send that rescuer to activate the emergency response system while you remain with the victim.	
5. Open the airway with a tongue-jaw lift. If you see the object, remove it *(no blind finger sweeps)*.	
6. Open the airway (head tilt–chin lift or jaw thrust), attempt rescue breathing; if no chest rise, reopen the airway (reposition head and chin) and try to ventilate again.	
7. If ventilation is unsuccessful, provide 5 abdominal thrusts with the victim supine (use proper hand position, avoiding the xiphoid).	
8. Repeat steps 5 through 7 until effective, then provide additional steps of CPR as needed.*	
9. If rescuer is alone and airway obstruction is not relieved after about 1 minute, activate the emergency response system.	

*If the victim is breathing or resumes normal breathing and no trauma is suspected, place in the recovery position.

Comments _____

_____

Instructor _____

Circle one: Complete   Needs more practice

Appendix B
BLS Performance Criteria

American Heart
Association®

*Learn and Live*SM

Healthcare Provider Skills Performance Sheet
Child FBAO in Unresponsive Victim
Performance Criteria

Participant Name _____ Date _____

Performance Guidelines	Performed
1. Establish unresponsiveness. If a second rescuer is available, send that rescuer to activate the emergency response system while you remain with the victim.	
2. Open the airway (head tilt–chin lift or jaw thrust) and check for breathing. If breathing is absent or inadequate, go to step 3.	
3. Attempt to ventilate; if unsuccessful (chest does not rise), reopen the airway (reposition head and chin) and try to ventilate again.	
4. If ventilation is unsuccessful, perform up to 5 abdominal thrusts with the victim supine (use proper hand position, avoid the xiphoid).	
5. Open the airway with a tongue-jaw lift. If you see the object, remove it *(no blind finger sweeps)*.	
6. Repeat steps 3 through 5 until ventilation is effective, then continue the steps of CPR as needed.*	
7. If rescuer is alone and airway obstruction is not relieved after about 1 minute, activate the emergency response system.	

*If the victim is breathing or resumes normal breathing and no trauma is suspected, place in the recovery position.

Comments _____

_____

_____

_____

_____

Instructor _____

Circle one: Complete   Needs more practice

Appendix B

BLS for Healthcare Provider Course
CPR and AED for Victims 1 to 8 Years of Age
Performance Criteria

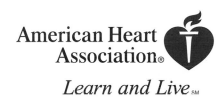

Participant Name _____ Date _____

Performance Guidelines	Performance	
CPR Skills	**Satisfactory**	**Remediate**
1. Establish unresponsiveness — direct coworker to activate the emergency response system and get the AED.		
2. Open the airway (head tilt–chin lift or, if trauma is suspected, jaw thrust) — check breathing (look, listen, and feel).		
3. If breathing is absent or inadequate, give 2 slow breaths (1 to 1½ seconds per breath) that cause the chest to rise (if chest does not rise, reposition, reattempt). Allow for adequate exhalation time.		
4. Check carotid pulse and other signs of circulation *(no signs of circulation).* Start chest compressions (ratio of 5 compressions to 1 breath at about 100 compressions per minute).		
AED Skills (AED arrives after CPR skills have been adequately assessed. Assume that 1 minute of CPR was provided.)		
5. Place the AED next to the victim. POWER ON the AED and note time.		
6. Attach electrode pads in the proper position (sternal-apex or as pictured on each of the AED electrodes) with proper contact and no overlap of pads.		
7. Clear the victim and press the ANALYZE button, if present. *(AED advises shock and charges electrodes.)*		
8. Clear the victim and press the SHOCK button, if advised. Stop timing for collapse-to-shock interval. (May repeat 1 to 2 more analyze-shock cycles. Stop when AED gives *"no shock indicated"* message.)		
9. Check carotid pulse and other signs of circulation. *(Pulse, breathing, coughing, movement present.)*		
10. Continue to monitor breathing and signs of circulation until advanced life support rescuers arrive. (If trauma is not suspected, place in a recovery position with AED attached.)		

(continued on next page)

CPR and AED Performance Criteria
for Victims 1 to 8 Years of Age (continued)

Critical Actions	Performance	
	Satisfactory	Remediate
• Assess responsiveness.		
• Activate the emergency response system (or send second rescuer); get the AED.		
• Open the airway, check breathing.		
• If breathing is absent or inadequate, provide 2 breaths (must cause chest to rise).		
• Check pulse and other signs of circulation.		
• Begin chest compressions (must have proper hand placement). Provide chest compressions and rescue breathing in a 5:1 ratio for 1 minute.		
• After 1 minute of CPR when AED arrives: POWER ON the AED.		
• Attach electrode pads to patient's bare chest in proper location with adequate skin contact and no overlap of pads.		
• "Clear" victim before ANALYZE and SHOCK.		
• Push SHOCK button (if not automated) to attempt defibrillation		
• Check breathing and signs of circulation after *"no shock indicated"* message.		
• Interval from collapse to first shock is less than 3 minutes, interval from AED arrival to first shock is less than 90 seconds		
• Rescuer should be prepared to continue CPR if nonshockable rhythm is present.		

Comments _____

Instructor _____

Circle one: Complete   Needs more practice

Appendix B
Performance Evaluation
BLS for Healthcare Providers Course

Integrated Adult FBAO and Rescue Breathing
Skills Performance Sheet

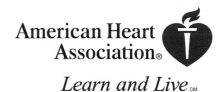

American Heart
Association®

Learn and Live SM

Instructions to Rescuer: You and a colleague enter a waiting room to find an adult man who appears to be in distress. He is clutching his throat. You have a mask or barrier device, but there is no other equipment in the room.

Participant Name _____ Date _____

Performance Guidelines *(Instructor cues to rescuers are in bold italics.)*	**Performed**
Responsive Victim	
1. Asks "Are you choking?" *(He nods yes.)* Asks "Can you speak?" *(He cannot speak.)* Tells the victim "I am going to help."	
2. Gives abdominal thrusts using the proper hand position (avoids the xiphoid). *(The victim is not pregnant or obese.)*	
3. Repeats thrusts until the foreign body is expelled or the victim becomes unresponsive. *(The foreign body is not expelled.)*	
Victim Becomes Unresponsive — Airway Remains Obstructed	
4. Eases the victim to the ground. Sends colleague to activate the emergency response system and bring the AED.	
5. Opens the airway with a tongue-jaw lift and looks for the object *(no object seen)*. Performs a finger sweep *(no object found)*.	
6. Opens the airway (head tilt–chin lift) and tries to ventilate *(chest does not rise)*. Repositions the head and tries to ventilate again *(chest does not rise)*.	
7. Performs 5 abdominal thrusts with the victim on his back (uses proper hand position, avoids the xiphoid).	
8. Opens the airway with a tongue-jaw lift and looks for the object *(object seen)*. Performs a finger sweep *(object removed)*.	
9. Opens the airway and attempts to provide 2 ventilations *(chest rises)*.	
10. Checks carotid pulse and other signs of circulation *(pulse present, no breathing)*.	
11. Performs mouth-to-mask (or barrier device) rescue breathing for several breaths.	
Colleague returns bringing a code cart with AED. The code team is on the way. Rescuers demonstrate each of the following skills for several breaths:	
12. One-rescuer bag-mask ventilation with oxygen.	
13. Two-rescuer bag-mask ventilation with oxygen. (One student is evaluated holding the mask in position with head tilt–chin lift and forming an effective seal while the second student compresses the bag.*)	
Victim Begins Breathing Normally	
14. Because there was no trauma, place the victim in the recovery position.	

*If there is only one student, instructor acts as colleague/Rescuer 2 and compresses the bag.

Comments _____

Instructor _____   **Circle one:**   Complete   Needs more practice

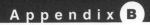

Appendix B
Performance Evaluation
BLS for Healthcare Providers Course

Integrated Infant FBAO, CPR, and Rescue Breathing
Skills Performance Sheet

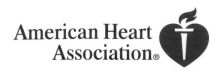

American Heart
Association®

Learn and Live ℠

Instructions to Rescuer: You and a colleague hear a call for help from the hospital cafeteria. You find a woman holding an infant who is clearly in distress. He is making frantic attempts to breathe and his face is turning blue, but he is making no noise. You suspect that he is choking. The cafeteria is equipped with a standard CPR kit, which includes pediatric barrier devices.

Participant Name _____ Date _____

Performance Guidelines *(Instructor cues to rescuers are in bold italics.)*	Performed
Responsive Victim	
1. Confirms severe or complete airway obstruction with poor air exchange, ineffective cough, and a weak cry. *(Infant is silent and trying to breathe.)*	
2. Gives up to 5 forceful back blows with the heel of hand while holding the infant in the correct position (face down over arm, the head supported and lower than the torso). *(The infant is still struggling silently; no object is expelled.)*	
3. Turns the infant face up in the correct position (face up over arm, the head supported and lower than the torso) and provides 5 chest thrusts using the 2-finger chest compression technique. *(The infant is still struggling silently; no object is expelled.)*	
4. Repeats 5 back blows followed by 5 chest thrusts until the object is expelled or infant becomes unresponsive. *(The object is not expelled; infant stops struggling and goes limp.)*	
Victim Becomes Unresponsive — Airway Remains Obstructed	
5. Sends colleague to activate the emergency response system.	
6. Opens the airway with a tongue-jaw lift, looks for the object, and removes it if seen *(no object seen—no blind finger sweeps)*.	
7. Opens the airway and attempts to provide a rescue breath *(chest does not rise)*. Repositions the head and tries to ventilate again *(chest does not rise)*.	
8. Provides 5 back blows, followed by 5 chest thrusts.	
9. Performs a tongue-jaw lift, looks for object, and removes it if seen *(object is seen and removed)*.	
10. Opens the airway using head tilt–chin lift or jaw thrust and attempts to provide 2 rescue breaths *(chest rises)*.	
11. Checks brachial pulse and other signs of circulation *(no signs of circulation)*.	
Airway Open. No Signs of Circulation *(Colleague has not yet returned.)*	
12. Begins cycles of 5 chest compressions (at least 100 compressions per minute) and 1 slow breath.	
13. After about 1 minute of rescue support, checks for signs of circulation *(pulse present)* and breathing *(breathing absent)*.	
Pulse Present — No Breathing	
14. Performs rescue breathing for several breaths (1 breath every 3 seconds for 4 to 6 breaths).	

Performance Guidelines	Performed
Colleague returns bringing an oxygen set-up with bag-mask device.	
15. Provides bag-mask ventilation with oxygen for several breaths.	
Colleague assesses the infant and finds a weak, slow pulse at a rate of 20 beats per minute.	
16. Performs 2-rescuer CPR using the 2-thumbs–encircled hands technique.	

Comments _____

Instructor _____

Circle one: Complete   Needs more practice

Appendix B
Performance Evaluation
BLS for Healthcare Providers Course

Integrated Child FBAO, CPR, and Rescue Breathing
Skills Performance Sheet

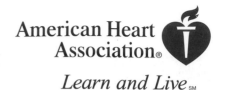

American Heart
Association®
Learn and Live sm

> **Instructions to Rescuer:** You and a colleague enter a waiting room and find a 4-year-boy who is responsive and appears to be in distress. He is clutching his throat. You have a mask or barrier device, but there is no other equipment in the room.

Participant Name _____ Date _____

Performance Guidelines *(Instructor cues to rescuers are in bold italics.)*	Performed
Responsive Victim	
1. Ask "Are you choking?" *(Child nods yes.)* Asks "Can you speak?" *(He cannot speak.)* Tells the child "I am going to help."	
2. Stands or kneels behind the child with arms encircling the child's abdomen. Gives abdominal thrusts using the proper hand position (avoids the xiphoid) and supports the body.	
3. Repeat thrusts until the object is expelled or the child becomes unresponsive *(object is not expelled).*	
Victim Becomes Unresponsive — Airway Remains Obstructed	
4. Lowers the child to the ground and sends colleague to activate the emergency response system and bring the AED.	
5. Opens the airway with a tongue-jaw lift. Looks for the object to remove it *(no object seen—no finger sweeps).*	
6. Opens the airway and attempts rescue breathing *(chest does not rise).* Reopens the airway with head tilt–chin lift (repositions head and chin) and tries to ventilate again *(chest does not rise).*	
7. Gives 5 abdominal thrusts with the victim on his back (uses proper hand position, avoids xiphoid).	
8. Performs a tongue-jaw lift, looks for the object, and removes it if seen *(object is seen and removed).*	
9. Opens the airway using head tilt–chin lift or jaw thrust and attempts to provide 2 rescue breaths *(chest rises).*	
No Signs of Circulation	
10. Checks carotid pulse and other signs of circulation *(no signs of circulation).*	
11. Begins cycles of 5 chest compressions (1-hand compression technique, about 100 compressions per minute) and 1 slow breath.	
12. After about 1 minute of CPR, checks for signs of circulation *(signs of circulation present)* and breathing *(breathing absent).*	
Pulse Present — No Breathing	
13. Performs rescue breathing for several breaths *(1 breath every 3 seconds for 4 to 6 breaths).*	

Performance Guidelines	Performed
Colleague returns bringing the AED and an oxygen set-up with bag-mask device. Rescuers demonstrate each of the following skills for several breaths:	
14. One-rescuer bag-mask ventilation with oxygen.	
15. Two-rescuer bag-mask ventilation with oxygen. (One student is evaluated holding the mask in position with head tilt–chin lift and forming an effective seal while the second student compresses the bag.*)	
Victim Begins Breathing Normally	
16. Because there was no trauma, rescuer places the victim in the recovery position.	

*If there is only one student, the instructor acts as colleague/Rescuer 2.

Comments _____

Instructor _____

Circle one: Complete   Needs more practice

Appendix B
Performance Evaluation
BLS for Healthcare Providers Course

Adult 1- and 2-Rescuer CPR With AED
Skills Performance Sheet

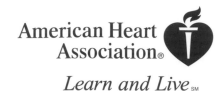

American Heart
Association®
Learn and Live sm

> **Instructions to Rescuer:** You and a colleague enter a room to find an adult man who appears to be unresponsive. There are no signs of trauma. You have a face mask or barrier device, but there is no other equipment in the room. The nearest AED is down the hall near the phone.

Participant Name _____ Date _____

Performance Guidelines *(Instructor cues to rescuers are in bold italics.)*	Performed
1. Checks responsiveness *(unresponsive).*	
2. Sends colleague to activate the emergency response system and get the AED.	
3. Opens the airway (head tilt–chin lift) and assesses for breathing (look, listen, and feel) *(no breathing).*	
4. Gives 2 slow breaths (2 seconds per breath) that cause the chest to rise. If the chest does not rise, reposition the head and try again *(chest rises).*	
5. Checks for carotid pulse and other signs of circulation *(no signs of circulation).*	
1-Rescuer CPR	
6. Starts 1-rescuer CPR at a ratio of 15 compressions to 2 ventilations.	
Colleague Arrives With AED	
7. Rescuer 1 continues with 1-rescuer CPR until directed to stop by Rescuer 2 (AED Rescuer).* Rescuer 2 places AED near the patient's head, turns it on (if necessary), and applies the electrodes. *(If the AED is fully automated, stay clear of the victim while the AED performs steps 8 and 9).*	
8. Follows AED prompts. If directed to press analyze, Rescuer 2 clears the victim and presses the analyze button.	
Shock Advised	
9. Follows AED prompts. If directed to provide a shock, Rescuer 2 clears the victim and presses the shock button. Then if so directed, analyzes again.	
AED Analyzes, No Shock Advised, No Signs of Circulation— 2-Rescuer CPR	
10. Rescuer 1 checks for a carotid pulse and other signs of circulation *(no signs of circulation).*	
11. Rescuers begin 2-rescuer CPR using the 15:2 compression-to-ventilation ratio. *Continue until AED signals a pause for analysis and assessment (no signs of circulation).*	
12. Code Team arrives and assumes care of the patient.	

*Note: If there is only 1 student, Rescuer 1 uses the AED and the instructor provides compressions during 2-rescuer CPR.

Comments _____

Instructor _____

Circle one: Complete   Needs more practice

Glossary

Abdominal thrust: A thrust applied to the abdomen just above the navel and well below the xiphoid to expel a foreign-body airway obstruction. Also called the Heimlich maneuver.

Active compression-decompression CPR (ACD-CPR): An alternative form of CPR using a hand-held mechanical device to augment chest relaxation between compressions. The device uses a type of suction cup attached to the chest. The device provides positive pressure to the chest on the compression downstroke and negative pressure to lift the anterior chest on the upstroke. Use of this device appears to augment venous return to the heart during CPR.

Acute coronary syndromes: A term that encompasses symptomatic conditions resulting in an inadequate blood supply to the heart, including angina and acute myocardial infarction.

Adhesive electrode pads: Pads that adhere directly to the skin of the patient's chest. These electrodes can be used to capture the surface ECG, and they can be used as a contact medium for conducting electric current from an automated external defibrillator (AED) or transcutaneous pacer to the patient.

Advance directive: A medical order written by a physician in response to the expressed wishes of the patient. The advance directive should state the level of care the patient desires at the end of life. An advance directive may name a surrogate decision maker to make those choices if the patient is unable to do so. In common usage this term includes living wills, but it is preferable that these terms are not interchanged. A living will contains an expression of the patient's wishes. An advance directive, in contrast, is a physician order that is based on the patient's wishes.

Advanced cardiovascular life support (ACLS): A group of interventions used to treat and stabilize adult victims of life-threatening cardiorespiratory emergencies and to resuscitate victims of cardiac arrest. These interventions include CPR, basic and advanced airway management, tracheal intubation, medications, electrical therapy, and intravenous (IV) access. ACLS also refers to a training course sponsored by the American Heart Association that instructs healthcare providers in the basic and advanced techniques of resuscitation.

Advocacy: Acting in the best interest of the patient.

Aerosol transmission: Transmission of disease by the inhalation of micro-organisms suspended in droplets in the air.

Agonal electrical cardiac activity: A cardiac arrest rhythm characterized by occasional wide complexes on the electrocardiogram (ECG).

Agonal respirations: Ineffective, reflex, gasping respiratory efforts that may occur at the moment of cardiac arrest.

Alveoli: Small, saclike outpouchings in the lungs where gas exchange takes place between alveolar gas and pulmonary capillary blood.

Amniotic fluid embolism: Arterial obstruction caused by amniotic fluid in the bloodstream.

Aneurysm: An abnormal localized dilation of a blood vessel wall, which weakens it, often causing sudden rupture and bleeding.

Angina: Transient pain, pressure, or discomfort resulting from a temporary lack of adequate blood supply to the heart muscle.

Antiplatelet agents: Platelets are small disc-shaped structures in the blood that adhere together or aggregate to form clots. Platelet aggregate activity serves an important function by stopping bleeding (hemostasis), but it also may contribute to the formation of harmful blood clots (thrombosis) in the coronary arteries or brain. Antiplatelet agents block this action. Aspirin is a well-known and effective antiplatelet agent.

Apneic: May refer to either a pause (of 20 seconds or longer) in breathing or complete cessation of breathing.

Arrhythmia: Abnormal heart rhythm.

Arteries: Muscular blood vessels that carry blood away from the heart.

Arterioles: Very small muscular blood vessels located throughout the body that regulate blood pressure.

Arteriosclerosis: Commonly called "hardening of the arteries," arteriosclerosis includes a variety of conditions that cause the artery walls to thicken and lose elasticity.

Asphyxia: A life-threatening condition caused by a lack of oxygen (ie, carbon monoxide poisoning).

Asymptomatic coronary artery disease (CAD): The phase of CAD in which the patient has not yet experienced symptoms.

Asystole: Cardiac standstill or an absence of any electrical cardiac rhythm; also called *flat line*.

Atherosclerosis: A process that leads to a group of diseases characterized by a thickening of artery walls. Atherosclerosis is a leading cause of death from heart attack and stroke.

Atrial fibrillation: An abnormal, irregular heart rhythm that results in quivering of the atria so that they no longer contract. This arrhythmia can lead to stasis of blood in the atria and formation of clots. These clots can embolize to other parts of the body.

Automated external defibrillator (AED): An external computerized defibrillator designed for use in unresponsive victims with no breathing and no signs of circulation. The AED captures the victim's ECG signal through adhesive electrodes placed on the victim's chest and analyzes the victim's heart rhythm, identifying shockable rhythms. Once a shockable rhythm is identified, the AED automatically charges to a preset energy level and provides voice prompts for the operator. When activated by the rescuer, the AED will deliver a shock through the adhesive electrodes.

Automaticity: The ability of cardiac tissue to generate its own electrical impulse.

Autonomy: The principle that a person should be free to make his or her own decisions.

Bag-mask (device): A mechanical aid used to deliver positive-pressure ventilation. The device consists of a bag with an oxygen inlet and a mask. Many bags contain a unidirectional valve to divert the patient's exhaled air into the atmosphere; a bag, unidirectional valve, and mask can be referred to as a bag-mask system.

Barrier device: Any number of devices used in rescue breathing (including face shields and masks) that create a physical barrier between a rescuer and a victim to decrease the small chance of disease transmission.

Basic life support (BLS): A group of actions and interventions used to treat, stabilize, and resuscitate victims of cardiac or respiratory arrest. These BLS actions and interventions include recognition of a cardiac or respiratory emergency or stroke, activation of the emergency response system, cardiopulmonary resuscitation (CPR), use of an AED, and relief of foreign-body airway obstruction. BLS also refers to a training course sponsored by the American Heart Association that instructs healthcare providers in the basic techniques of resuscitation.

Beneficence: The principle of doing good.

Biphasic: Having 2 phases or variations.

Biphasic waveform defibrillator: A defibrillator that delivers a current that flows in a positive direction for a specified duration and then reverses and flows in a negative direction for the remaining milliseconds of electrical discharge.

Bradycardia: Slow heart rate (usually less than 60 beats per minute in an adult).

Capillaries: Minute, thin-walled blood vessels in which there is an interchange of various substances between the blood and tissue, including gases.

Cardiac arrest: The cessation of a functional heartbeat.

Cardiopulmonary resuscitation: In the broadest sense, attempting any maneuvers or techniques designed to restore circulation, or a technique combining artificial ventilation and chest compressions designed to perfuse vital organs or restore circulation to a victim of cardiopulmonary arrest.

Cardiovascular: Pertaining to the heart and blood vessels.

Cardioversion: Typically referred to as synchronized cardioversion. This is the delivery of a shock to the heart in an attempt to terminate a rapid supraventricular arrhythmia. Cardioversion uses lower energy than defibrillation. Unlike defibrillation, the shock used for cardioversion is *timed* to coincide with the patient's R wave.

Cerebral: A term referring to the cerebrum, the main portion of the brain occupying the upper part of the cranial cavity.

Cerebral thrombosis: Formation of a blood clot in an artery in the brain. This is a common cause of an ischemic stroke.

Cerebrovascular: A term referring to the brain and the vessels that supply the brain with blood.

Chain of Survival: An American Heart Association metaphor that uses the links in a chain to describe the actions needed to save a victim of sudden cardiac arrest. The links in the adult Chain of Survival are early access to 911, early CPR, early defibrillation, and early advanced care. The links in the pediatric Chain of Survival are prevention of injury and arrest, early CPR, early access to 911, and early advanced care.

Cholesterol: A fatlike substance in the blood that contributes to the formation of atherosclerosis.

Cincinnati Stroke Scale: A focused physical exam designed to rapidly detect patients with stroke. This scale is designed to detect facial droop, arm drift (the patient's eyes are closed and the arms held out), and abnormal speech.

Computed tomography (CT) scan: A series of x-rays (radiographs) that are analyzed and reconstructed by a computer into a pictorial image of a part of the body. CT scans can be used to visualize a variety of disorders, including tumors, hemorrhages, and abscesses, and they may reveal areas of abnormal blood flow or injury. A CT scan of the brain is required to rule out the presence of hemorrhagic stroke before administration of fibrinolytics.

Coronary artery disease (CAD): A group of diseases, including angina and myocardial infarction, caused by the development of arteriosclerotic plaques that narrow the artery walls and obstruct distal blood flow to part of the heart.

Coronary artery spasm: Severe, usually localized constriction of a coronary artery resulting in a lack of blood supply to the heart.

Coronary care unit: A specialized intensive care unit in a hospital that treats victims of heart disease during the critical or unstable phase of their illness.

Coronary reperfusion: Restoration of some blood flow to an area of the heart. This may be accomplished by administration of fibrinolytics, angioplasty with or without stent placement, or coronary revascularization (coronary artery bypass grafting).

Coronary revascularization: The restoration of blood flow to the heart by means of blood vessel grafting.

Cricothyroidotomy (cricothyrotomy): A surgical procedure opening the cricothyroid membrane (in the windpipe of the neck) to provide an airway.

Critical incident stress debriefing (CISD): A group meeting of rescuers involved in a resuscitation attempt designed to educate and to ease the psychological and emotional impact of the incident.

Cyanosis: Bluish discoloration of the skin (most often around the lips and nail beds) caused by a severe lack of oxygen in the blood.

Deciliter: One tenth of a liter.

Defibrillation: The untimed (asynchronous) depolarization of the myocardium that *successfully* terminates ventricular fibrillation (VF) or pulseless ventricular tachycardia (VT). In defibrillation and defibrillation attempts, a shock is delivered to the myocardium, most often through the chest wall (although internal defibrillation may be accomplished if the chest is open). The goal of defibrillation is to enable resumption of a perfusing rhythm, but the shock may convert the rhythm to asystole. In common usage the term *defibrillation* is used interchangeably with the term *shock*. However, the shock is used to *attempt* defibrillation, and the term *defibrillation* should be reserved for the successful termination of VF/VT.

Defibrillator: A device used to deliver a shock to the heart. A defibrillation shock depolarizes the heart in an effort to suppress ventricular fibrillation (VF) or pulseless ventricular tachycardia (VT) and allow a perfusing rhythm to return. Defibrillators may be manual or automated (see Automated external defibrillator). Manual defibrillators often have the capacity to perform synchronized cardioversion (see Cardioversion).

Diabetes: A general term referring to persistent elevations of blood sugar in the bloodstream.

DNR (No CPR, DNAR): The terms *DNR ("do not resuscitate")*, *No CPR*, and *DNAR ("do not attempt resuscitation")* are used to indicate that in the event of a cardiac arrest, no cardiopulmonary resuscitative measures should be instituted.

Durable power of attorney for health care: An advance directive naming another person to make healthcare decisions if a patient is unable to do so.

Electrical therapy: Interventions used to convert, resuscitate, or stabilize a cardiac rhythm, including defibrillation, cardioversion, and pacing.

Embolic stroke: A stroke caused by an embolism.

Embolism: The sudden blockage of an artery by a clot, that has traveled through the bloodstream from another location.

Emergency cardiovascular care (ECC): A system including all interventions to manage emergencies related to the heart, blood vessels, and brain. These interventions include BLS, PALS, and ACLS assessments and interventions performed by bystanders, trained responders, healthcare professionals, and allied health personnel.

Emergency medical dispatchers (EMDs): EMS personnel who answer 911 calls and dispatch EMS responders to the scene of an emergency. EMDs also provide telephone instructions to bystanders at the scene while the responders are en route.

Emergency medical services (EMS): The planned configuration of community resources and personnel designed to respond to medical emergencies and provide immediate care to persons who have suffered an unexpected illness or injury. The EMS system includes EMS dispatchers and EMS responders.

Emergency medical technicians (EMTs): Prehospital emergency care providers trained in a program using the structure and guidelines set forth by the Department of Transportation (DOT).

EMS responders: A group of EMTs-basic, EMTs-intermediate, and EMTs-paramedic who respond with specialized equipment and resources to emergencies in the community.

Enhanced 911: An emergency medical dispatch system (911) that allows the dispatcher to identify the location and telephone number of incoming telephone calls. This system allows the dispatcher to send responders to the scene of an emergency even if the caller cannot provide the address or other information.

Epiglottis: A lidlike structure attached to the base of the tongue overhanging the entrance to the larynx. This structure normally prevents food from entering the larynx.

Epiglottitis: Inflammation (usually with swelling) of the epiglottis. This inflammation can lead to severe upper airway obstruction, particularly in young children who have relatively small upper airways.

Evidence based: The conscientious, explicit, and judicious use of current best medical and scientific evidence in determining recommendations for medical care or policy or decisions about patient care.

Exsanguination: Drainage or massive loss of blood from the body.

Face shield: A barrier device placed over the mouth and nose of a cardiac arrest victim (or manikin) during rescue breathing.

Fat emboli: Arterial obstruction caused by fat droplets in the bloodstream (usually the result of long bone fractures).

Fibrinolytic: A term referring to "clot-busting" medications administered to heart attack and stroke victims. If given within the recommended time, these drugs dissolve the blood clot that is causing the heart attack or stroke. The benefit of these medications is time-dependent.

First responders: A group including police officers and firefighters trained in a nationally recognized program to respond to emergencies with resources such as oxygen and an AED.

Focal neurologic dysfunction: Loss of function of part of the body caused by localized damage to the brain controlling that area.

Foreign-body airway obstruction (FBAO): An obstruction of the airway in any location from the mouth to the bronchioles, caused by food, toys, or other external objects.

Genetic: Related to heredity.

Glasgow Coma Scale: A reliable scale used to quickly assess the severity of neurologic dysfunction in patients with altered consciousness. The scale is based on the best responses for eye opening (1 to 4), verbal responses (1 to 5), and movement (1 to 6). The total score ranges from 3 to 15.

Good Samaritan laws: Laws (which vary from state to state) that generally protect a person who renders emergency aid from civil damages if the person acts in good faith and not for remuneration.

HDL: High-density lipoprotein ("good" cholesterol).

Heimlich maneuver: An abdominal thrust performed in children or adults (not infants) to relieve FBAO.

Hemorrhagic stroke: Localized brain damage caused by bleeding resulting from the rupture of a blood vessel in the brain.

Hemothorax: Bleeding within the pleural cavity (the space between the lung and chest wall).

Hyperbaric oxygen chamber: A compartment capable of delivering oxygen at pressures many times higher than barometric pressure. Hyperbaric oxygen may be used to treat carbon monoxide poisoning, decompression sickness, and anaerobic infections.

Hypercholesterolemia: High levels of cholesterol in the bloodstream.

Hypertension: High blood pressure. Systolic pressure, diastolic pressure, or both may be elevated.

Hypertriglyceridemia: High levels of triglycerides (fats) in the bloodstream.

Hypoglycemia: Low blood sugar.

Hypothermia: An abnormally low body temperature caused by exposure to environmental extremes or physiological factors that affect mechanisms of heat production and heat loss.

Hypothermic: Referring to a low body temperature.

Hypovolemia: Low blood volume caused by hemorrhage, burns, metabolic disorders, or other causes of loss of body fluid. Hypovolemia may be absolute (caused by intravascular volume loss) or relative (caused by expansion of the vascular space)

Hypoxia: Reduced oxygen supply (delivery) to the body's tissues. When hypoxia is present, tissues must switch to anaerobic metabolism, and lactic acid is generated (lactic acidosis).

Implanted cardioverter defibrillator (ICD): A biomedical device (slightly larger than a pacemaker) implanted under the skin of the chest or upper abdomen and joined to the heart by wire electrodes. An ICD detects abnormal ("shockable") heart rhythms (ventricular tachycardia or fibrillation) and automatically defibrillates the heart if required.

Incontinence: Loss of urinary or bowel control.

Infectious disease: A classification of disease in which the causative agent can be transmitted from one person to another directly or indirectly.

Interposed abdominal compression CPR (IAC-CPR): A 2- or 3-person CPR technique that includes manual compression of the abdomen during the relaxation phase of chest compression. This alternative form of in-hospital CPR requires an additional rescuer to press on the abdomen in the midline, halfway between the xiphoid process and the umbilicus.

Intracerebral hemorrhage: Bleeding into brain tissue caused by rupture of a blood vessel. Hypertension is the most common cause of intracerebral hemorrhage.

Intravascular: Within the blood vessels.

Ischemia: Inadequate blood supply to an organ such as the heart or brain.

Ischemic stroke: Localized brain damage caused by blockage of a blood vessel supplying the brain. A blood clot is the most common cause of blood vessel blockage. The blood clot may form at the site of the blockage (thrombotic stroke) or originate elsewhere in the body (usually the heart) and travel to the blood vessel in the brain (embolic stroke).

Justice: The principle of fairness in the allocation of resources and the physician's obligation to patients.

Laryngeal edema: Swelling of the larynx and surrounding tissues. This swelling can result in airway obstruction.

Laryngospasm: Severe constriction of the larynx.

Larynx: The structure in the neck formed by rings of cartilage guarding the entrance to the trachea and functioning secondarily as the organ of voice. Commonly called the *voice box.*

LDL: Low-density lipoprotein ("bad" cholesterol).

Living will: An expression of an individual's wishes regarding healthcare issues at the end of life. It should be enforced by a formal advance directive that comes from a physician.

Los Angeles Prehospital Stroke Screen (LAPSS): A focused physical exam designed to quickly identify patients with stroke.

Medullary respiratory center: The portion of the medulla in the brainstem that is responsible for monitoring and controlling respiration.

Microorganisms: Microscopic organisms, including bacteria, fungi, and viruses.

Mobile life support unit: An intensive care transport vehicle that treats victims of a wide variety of illnesses and injuries using specialized equipment and personnel.

Modifiable: Changeable.

Monomorphic: Existing in only 1 form.

Monophasic: Exhibiting only 1 phase or variation.

Morphology: Form and structure.

Mouth-to-nose ventilation: An alternative form of rescue breathing in which the rescuer provides positive-pressure ventilation through the victim's nose. This technique is recommended when it is impossible to ventilate through the victim's mouth, when the mouth cannot be opened, or when a tight mouth-to-mouth seal is difficult to achieve.

Myocardial infarction (MI): Death of heart tissue commonly caused by a blockage of a coronary artery owing to an arteriosclerotic plaque, thrombus, embolus, or spasm.

Myocardial ischemia: Inadequate delivery of oxygen to the heart muscle. This ischemia may create pain, called *angina*.

Needle cricothyroidotomy (needle cricothyrotomy): Placement of a needle through the cricothyroid membrane (in the windpipe) to provide an airway. This is used as a temporary measure (by a trained and qualified rescuer) until a foreign object can be removed or a cricothyroidotomy can be performed.

Neurologic dysfunction: Abnormal function caused by neurologic insult or injury.

Nicotine: A poisonous, colorless chemical obtained from tobacco.

Nonmaleficence: The principle that encompasses the ethical principle of "first do no harm."

Normothermic: Normal core body temperature.

Percutaneous coronary interventions (PCIs): A variety of cardiac procedures using a catheter in combination with other devices to open a blocked coronary artery and maintain patency. PCIs include angioplasty and stent placement.

Percutaneous transluminal coronary angioplasty (PTCA): The process of clearing a blocked coronary artery with a balloon that dilates and compresses an arteriosclerotic plaque against the artery wall.

Pericardial tamponade: A collection of blood or fluid in the pericardial sac around the heart, which can impair cardiac function and obstruct venous return to the heart.

Peripartum: Pertaining to the period immediately before, during, and after the birth of a baby.

Pharynx: The musculomembranous area between the mouth and nares and the esophagus. It communicates with the esophagus, the larynx, the mouth, the nasal passages, and the auditory tubes.

Platelets: Disc-shaped structures in the blood that aggregate (stick together or adhere) to stop bleeding. These platelets can exert a protective effect because they protect from bleeding (hemostasis), but they can also contribute to clot formation (thrombosis) that can lead to myocardial infarction or ischemic stroke.

Pneumatic antishock garment (PASG): Pneumatic trousers used to control hemorrhage in the legs and pelvis, thereby increasing peripheral vascular resistance.

Pneumatic vest CPR: An alternative form of CPR using an inflatable vest that fits completely around the patient's chest. The vest cyclically inflates and deflates, producing an increase in intrathoracic pressure.

Pocket mask: A device that consists of a mask and 1-way valve used to give rescue breaths and provide a physical barrier between the rescuer and the victim.

Polymorphic: Existing in more than 1 form.

Positive-pressure ventilation: The act of delivering air into the lungs under pressure (ie, bag-mask ventilation).

Postmenopausal: Occurring after menopause (cessation of menstruation in the female, usually by the age of 48 to 50).

Prearrival instructions: Instructions given by a dispatcher to a layperson at the scene of an emergency before the arrival of EMS. Instructions may include how to perform chest compressions and rescue breathing, how to assist with childbirth, etc.

Primary hypertension (essential hypertension): High blood pressure of unknown cause.

Primary prevention: A number of changes in behavior or lifestyle designed to prevent disease or injury.

Psychomotor: Pertaining to physical actions, which are the end result of mental activity.

Public access defibrillation (PAD): A healthcare initiative sponsored by the American Heart Association and other organizations that places AEDs throughout the community in the hands of trained lay rescuers. The goal of PAD programs is to shorten the interval between collapse due to sudden cardiac arrest and defibrillation. This should improve survival from sudden cardiac arrest.

Pulmonary embolism: An embolism that causes arterial obstruction in the lung.

Pulseless electrical activity (PEA): A cardiac arrest rhythm characterized by organized electrical activity of the heart but without a palpable pulse.

Quality assurance: An ongoing process of continuous evaluation and assessment of a program with feedback of information to participants. The purpose is to maintain and continually improve quality in the service delivered.

Recurrent VF: Ventricular fibrillation that occurs again.

Refibrillation: The reoccurrence of VF after conversion to an organized rhythm.

Regurgitation: To vomit partially digested food. This term can also be used to indicate backward flow of blood, such as occurs from the left ventricle to the left atrium through an insufficient mitral valve.

Reperfusion: The process of restoring blood flow to a tissue bed. Coronary reperfusion can involve techniques such as fibrinolysis (use of "clot-busters") or angioplasty. Reperfusion can also occur when circulation is restored (eg, to the brain) following cardiac arrest.

Respiratory arrest: Cessation of breathing.

Respiratory failure: The state that exists when the respiratory system can no longer support life. If an intervention is not provided, the victim will become progressively more hypoxic or hypercarbic, or both, and will ultimately die.

Respiratory insufficiency: Respiratory function that is inadequate to maintain normal levels of oxygen and carbon dioxide in the blood.

Secondary hypertension: High blood pressure caused by a condition such as kidney disease.

Secondary prevention: Actions taken to prevent further complications after an injury or illness.

Silent ischemia: An instance in which a patient experiences an ischemic event in the absence of chest pain, making diagnosis of acute MI more difficult. Women, persons with diabetes, and the elderly are more prone to silent ischemia than others.

Stroke: A disruption in blood supply to a region of the brain that causes acute neurologic impairment.

Stroke Chain of Survival and Recovery: The term used to describe the actions for survival and recovery from stroke, which are (1) early recognition, (2) early activation of the EMS system and dispatch instruction, and (3) early EMS response, treatment, and transport.

Subarachnoid hemorrhage: Bleeding into the surface of the brain caused by rupture of a blood vessel. The most common cause of a subarachnoid hemorrhage is rupture of a cerebral aneurysm.

Subdiaphragmatic: A term indicating the area below the diaphragm (the muscular partition separating the abdominal and thoracic cavities).

Sudden cardiac arrest: Sudden or unexpected cessation of heart function, most often caused by a sudden arrhythmia, such as VF or pulseless VT.

Suffocation: Cessation of respiration, most often resulting from obstruction to air flow, such as occurs with obstruction to air passages in victims of avalanche.

Supine: A term used to describe someone who is lying down with the face upward.

Supraventricular tachycardia (SVT): An abnormally rapid cardiac rhythm generated from an electrical focus in the heart that is above the ventricles. SVT typically produces a heart rate greater than 140 beats per minute in the adult and greater than 180 to 220 beats per minute in the infant or child.

Syncope: A temporary loss of consciousness due to cerebral ischemia.

Tension pneumothorax: Air trapped in the pleural space (the space between the lung and the chest wall) caused by a 1-way valve effect. A tension pneumothorax results in increased intrathoracic pressure, respiratory failure, decreased blood return to the heart, and shock.

Tidal volume: Volume of air inspired and expired during 1 respiratory cycle; normal tidal volume at rest is 500 mL.

Tracheobronchial: Pertaining to the trachea (windpipe) or bronchi within the lung.

Tracheostomy: The surgical creation of an opening into the trachea through the neck.

Transient ischemic attack (TIA): A reversible episode of focal neurologic dysfunction.

Transthoracic impedance: The resistance to transmission of electrical current represented by the skin, fat, muscle, and lung of a patient's chest.

Tympanic membrane: The eardrum.

Universal choking sign: The sign in which a victim clutches his neck with both hands, indicating a foreign-body airway obstruction.

Universal precautions: Steps taken to prevent potential contact with body substances that may carry the human immunodeficiency virus (HIV) or hepatitis B virus (HBV). This approach is designed to prevent the transmission of disease by using gloves, goggles, masks, and gowns.

Utstein style: A method of data collection that includes a uniform definition of terms and time intervals related to the discovery, assessment, and management of prehospital and in-hospital cardiac arrest. The Utstein guidelines have been developed to guide collection, publication, and comparison of data in human and laboratory resuscitation research.

Veins: Blood vessels that return blood to the heart.

Vena cava: The largest vein in the body, which returns blood to the right side of the heart.

Ventricular fibrillation (VF): A chaotic and disorganized heart rhythm that results in cardiac arrest.

Ventricular tachycardia (VT): An abnormally rapid heart rhythm generated within the ventricles. VT by itself or by its degeneration into VF can result in cardiac arrest.

Waveform: The form and structure of an electrically conducted impulse.

Xiphoid process: The bony protuberance at the base of the sternum.